YOUR PHARMACIST'S GUIDE TO
SAVING MONEY AND STAYING HEALTHY

UNLOCK COST SAVINGS, ESSENTIAL
MEDICATION ADVICE, NATURAL REMEDIES,
AND NAVIGATING HEALTHCARE WITH EASE

Dr. Rhowela A. Friel, PharmD

DISCLAIMER

This book, "Your Pharmacist's Guide to Saving Money and Staying Healthy," all its contents, is provided for informational purposes only. The author and the publisher make no representations or guarantees on the content's completeness, accuracy, applicability, or fitness found within. The information contained in this book is not intended to serve as a replacement for professional medical advice, diagnosis, or treatment. Readers are advised to consult a licensed healthcare professional for any concerns regarding their health or medications before starting, changing, or discontinuing any health or medication regimen.

The author and publisher thus explicitly disclaim any responsibility for any harm, loss, or risk—personal or otherwise—that may arise from using or putting any of the information in this book to use. Any names of medications, products, or brands mentioned are used only for illustrative purposes and do not imply endorsement. The trademarks and brand names belong to their respective owners and are acknowledged within the book. The mention of these brand names and trademarks does not constitute an infringement of intellectual property rights.

By reading this book, you acknowledge that there will be no recourse against the author or the publisher for any kind of damages—direct, indirect, consequential, special, exemplary, or otherwise—resulting from its use. The information in this book is based on the author's professional experience and knowledge up to the publication date. It is subject to change based on ongoing research and development in the medical field.

To ensure this book is used as intended, understand that it is for educational purposes only and not a substitute for professional medical advice. Please consult a healthcare professional for personal health concerns. The information herein is offered "as is" without warranties, and using it is at your own risk. Discontinuation of use is advised if you disagree with these terms.

Copyright © 2024 Rhowela A. Friel
All rights reserved.

DEDICATION

To my husband—thank you for always believing in me, especially when I struggled to believe in myself. Your quiet support and steady love helped bring this book to life.

To our girls—you are my reason, my joy, and the heart behind every page.

And to you—if you're holding this book, know that it was written for you. For the questions you're carrying, the care you're giving, and the strength you don't always see. I'm so glad you're here.

WELCOME

Before you get started, I just wanted to say thank you—for picking up this book, for caring enough to look for answers, and for being the kind of person who shows up when it matters.

I also wanted to let you know I've built a space online to keep the support going: rhowelaafriel.com.

It's where I share what I've learned (and keep learning) as a pharmacist, a mom, and someone who knows how overwhelming care can feel sometimes. You'll find free resources, gentle tools, and updates on what's coming next. No noise, no pressure—just what might actually help.

And if this book made things a little clearer or calmer for you? Leaving a quick review helps others find their way here too.

I'm so grateful you're here.

TABLE OF CONTENTS

PREFACE 11

HOW TO USE THIS BOOK 13

CHAPTER 1: EXPLORING THE PHARMACY WORLD 15

    1.1: Meet the Pharmacy Team   15
    1.2: Types of Pharmacies Explained   17
    1.3: The Journey of a Prescription   18
    1.4: Refills and Their Rules   20
    1.5: Prescription Validity Insights   23
    1.6: Transfer Process Uncovered   25
    1.7: Out-of-Stock Solutions   27
    1.8: Backorder Strategies   29
    1.9: Pharmacy's Role in Healthcare   30

CHAPTER 2: UNDERSTANDING MEDICATIONS 35

    2.1: Decoding Medication Labels   35
    2.2: Importance of Medication Adherence   36
    2.3: Managing Side Effects   38
    2.4: Medication Interactions Simplified   40

CHAPTER 3: MEDICATION MANAGEMENT
MASTERY 45

    3.1: Administering Medications Correctly   45
    3.2: Managing Complex Regimens   48
    3.3: Dealing with Missed Doses   50
    3.4: Techniques for Pill Swallowing   52
    3.5: Mitigating Side Effects   54
    3.6: Risk of Expired Medications   56

CHAPTER 4: INSURANCE NAVIGATION 63

- 4.1: Health Insurance Basics — 63
- 4.2: Prior Authorizations Explained — 65
- 4.3: Insurance Formularies and Cost Savings — 66
- 4.4: Understanding Primary vs. Secondary Insurance — 68
- 4.5: Appeals Process and Patient Rights — 69
- 4.6: Medication Refunds and Rights — 70

CHAPTER 5: SAVING MONEY ON MEDICATIONS 73

- 5.1: Generic vs. Brand-Name Drugs — 73
- 5.2: Finding the Best Pharmacy Deals — 74
- 5.3: Discount, Coupons, and Assistance Programs — 76
- 5.4: Discussing Alternative Medications — 77

CHAPTER 6: GOVERNMENT HEALTH PROGRAMS 81

- 6.1: Medicare, Medicaid, CHIP, and VA Overview — 81
- 6.2: State Pharma-ceutical Assistance Programs — 85
- 6.3: The 340B Drug Pricing Program — 86

CHAPTER 7: OVER-THE-COUNTER (OTC) MEDICATIONS 91

- 7.1: Understanding OTC Medications — 91
- 7.2 Key Considerations for OTC Use — 92
- 7.3: OTC Remedies for Common Issues — 93
- 7.4: Consulting Healthcare Professionals — 101

CHAPTER 8: NATURAL AND HERBAL REMEDIES 105

- 8.1 Using Herbal Remedies Safely — 105
- 8.2: Remedies for Common Health Issues — 107
- 8.3: Home Remedies and DIY Solutions — 113

CHAPTER 9: DIETARY INTERACTIONS WITH MEDICATIONS 119

- 9.1: Nutritional Impacts on Medications — 119
- 9.2: Food and Medication Interactions — 120
- 9.3: Dietary Management Tips — 122

CHAPTER 10: PEDIATRIC MEDICATION MANAGEMENT 127

- 10.1: Treating Common Childhood Conditions — 127
- 10.2: Allergies vs. Cold and Flu — 137
- 10.3: Pediatric Dosing and Administration — 140
- 10.4: Medication Adherence in Children — 141

CHAPTER 11: ELDERLY MEDICATION MANAGEMENT 145

- 11.1: Managing Medications for the Elderly — 145
- 11.2: Treatments for Elderly Ailments — 147
- 11.3 Tailored Medication Choices for the Elderly — 157
- 11.4: The Beers List Explained — 158
- 11.5: Opioids and Benzodiazepines — 159

CHAPTER 12: MEDICATIONS DURING PREGNANCY AND NURSING 167

- 12.1: Pregnancy Category Insights — 167
- 12.2: Prenatal Vitamin Guide — 169
- 12.3: Safe Treatments for Common Ailments — 170
- 12.4: Considerations for Pregnant and Nursing Women — 179

CHAPTER 13: SAFE MEDICATION PRACTICES 185

13.1: Understanding Safe Practices — 185
13.2: Dosage and Timing Importance — 188
13.3: Risks of Medication Sharing — 190
13.4: Medication Recall Procedures — 191

CHAPTER 14: MEDICATION STORAGE AND DISPOSAL 195

14.1: Proper Storage Techniques — 195
14.2: Safe Disposal of Medications — 197
14.3: Sharps Disposal Guidelines — 200

CHAPTER 15: TRAVELING WITH MEDICATIONS 205

15.1: Travel Preparation — 205
15.2: Airport Security Tips — 207
15.3: Time Zone Adjustments — 208
15.4: Emergency Medication Strategies — 210

CHAPTER 16: VACCINATIONS AND YOUR HEALTH 215

16.1: Vaccination Process in Pharmacies — 215
16:2: Common Vaccinations — 218
16.3: Vaccine Importance — 220
16.4: Travel Vaccines — 223
16.5: Free Vaccine Resources — 224

CHAPTER 17: LAB TEST AND MEDICATION IMPACT 229

- 17.1: Common Lab Tests — 229
- 17.2: Interpreting Lab Results — 231
- 17.3: Medication Effects on Lab Results — 233
- 17.4: Medication and Lab Test Management — 235

CHAPTER 18: PHARMACY FAQS AND TROUBLESHOOTING 239

- 18.1: Pharmacy Policies and Procedures — 239
- 18.2: Answering Common Questions — 244
- 18.3: Practical Problem-Solving Tips — 255

CONCLUSION 263

ACKNOWLEDGMENTS 265

ABOUT THE AUTHOR 267

ADDITIONAL RESOURCES 269

PREFACE

Hi there—I'm really glad you picked up this book.

I'm a pharmacist, a mom, and someone who's spent over a decade helping people figure out medications, make sense of symptoms, and feel more confident about the care they're giving (or getting). Through the years, I've had thousands of conversations at the pharmacy counter—and I've seen just how often the same questions come up.

"How do I know this is safe?"
"What's the difference between all these labels?"
"Should I call the doctor, or can I handle this at home?"

That's why I wrote this book.

It's not meant to replace your provider or give you all the answers—but to offer something steady and practical when things feel unclear. Something you can flip through when you're tired, overwhelmed, or just want to double-check what's okay to try.

Inside, you'll find pharmacist-approved info, practical tips, and natural remedies—all explained in a clear, no-pressure way. Think of it like chatting with someone who's been there and just wants to help make things a little easier.

We'll cover everything from what to keep in your medicine cabinet to how to use herbal support safely. You'll also find tips for reading medication labels, talking to providers, and navigating pharmacy visits with a little more ease.

No fancy language. No complicated routines. Just useful, real-world support you can turn to when someone's not feeling well—or when you're trying to stay ahead of things.

Thanks for being here. I hope this book becomes something you come back to—not just for information, but for reassurance, too.

HOW TO USE THIS BOOK

Welcome—I'm really glad you're here.

This book was made to be easy to use, especially on days when you're feeling tired, unsure, or just need a little extra support. Think of it like a guide you can flip through when something's off and you want to figure out what might help.

Start with what brought you here.
Maybe you've got questions about what to try, how to save money, or if that home remedy is actually worth it. You'll find real answers here—backed by research, explained in plain language, and grounded in what's practical.

Flip to what you need.
You don't have to read this cover to cover (though you totally can!). Each section stands on its own, so feel free to jump to whatever fits—headaches, sleep support, sore throats, or DIY care. Use the Table of Contents like a menu.

Keep an eye out for helpful tips.
You'll see notes, reminders, and ideas I've shared with patients, friends, and my own family—simple things that can actually help. They're easy to spot as you read.

Keep it close.
Tuck it next to your medicine basket, in your kitchen, or wherever you tend to reach when something's off. This book is meant to work in real life—so make it yours.

Share what helps.
If something in here makes the day feel a little easier, pass it on. A calming tea or quick tip can be just the thing someone else needs too.

You don't have to remember it all. Just come back when you need steady support that actually makes sense.

CHAPTER 1:
EXPLORING THE PHARMACY WORLD

Welcome to the exciting world of pharmacy, where science and customer service unite to keep you healthy. I'm here to guide you through the diverse landscape of pharmacies, from the bustling neighborhood stores to the advanced hospital dispensaries, each with its vital role in healthcare. In this chapter, I'll take you behind the scenes to uncover how a piece of paper from your doctor becomes the medicine in your hands. We'll uncover the process of getting prescription refills, transferring prescriptions, and handling situations when medications are out of stock. You'll also discover how we manage backorders and why pharmacists are a crucial link in the healthcare chain. Get ready to explore the essential yet often overlooked operations of the pharmacy world, bringing clarity to every step of your medication journey.

1.1: Meet the Pharmacy Team

Allow me to take you behind the scenes of our pharmacy community. Consider us a team dedicated to providing you with the greatest care and service possible, whether you're picking up a prescription or simply seeking medical advice. Here's a quick list of who does what.

Pharmacists:
That's folks like me! We're your go-to for all things medication. We not only verify that your medications are filled correctly, but we also offer guidance

on how to take them safely, manage any adverse effects, and answer any health-related questions you may have. Need info on vitamins or thinking about getting a flu shot? We're here for that, too.

Pharmacy Technicians:
Consider these individuals to be key parts of our pharmacy machine. They manage the technical aspects, from data entry to dealing with insurance companies. They play a significant role in ensuring that your medication is properly prepared and delivered on time.

Pharmacy Clerks:
These are probably the first friendly faces you'll encounter. Our clerks make sure everything runs properly for you from the time you walk in. They take care of billing and walk you through the checkout procedure. Do you want to drop off a prescription or ask a quick question? They are ready to assist.

Pharmacy Interns:
These future pharmacists, currently students, are with us to study everything about the pharmacy profession. They're involved in deeper aspects like medication management and patient education, offering fresh, knowledgeable insights to help you manage your health.

Pharmacy Externs:
Similar to interns, but with a concentration on developing the technical skills required to be a pharmacy technician. They're in the thick of learning how to dispense medications efficiently, manage stock, and deliver exceptional customer service. This real-world exposure is critical for their growth as future pharmacy technicians.

Our pharmacy team is a close-knit group of experts, each with a unique role and a shared commitment to your health and well-being. From pharmacists to technicians, clerks, interns, and externs, we all work together, leveraging our individualized and thorough expertise to provide you with the best care possible. Next time you visit, feel free to ask questions or just say hi. We're here to support you every step of the way on your health journey.

1.2: Types of Pharmacies Explained

Pharmacies play an important role in the ever-changing world of healthcare that goes beyond just dispensing medications. Let me guide you through the diverse types of pharmacies, each tailored to meet specific healthcare needs.

Retail Pharmacies:
These are your go-to locations for quick refills and health needs. They can be found in locations like your local grocery or corner shop and are ideal for picking up medications, getting health advice, or even getting a flu vaccine. They are the friendly face of pharmacy care, always available when you need a brief consultation or a band-aid.

Specialty Pharmacies:
Do you have something a bit more complicated than a cold? Specialty pharmacies tackle the difficult stuff—think drugs for chronic illnesses like multiple sclerosis or unusual ailments that require a little more attention than what you'd find on the shelf. They function similarly to personal health coaches, providing individualized support and ensuring that your treatment is appropriate.

Compounding Pharmacies:
Imagine a pharmacy that functions similarly to a chef's kitchen, creating personalized prescriptions particularly for you. Do you require a lower dosage? Are you allergic to any common ingredients? They can adjust your medications to meet your specific needs. It's an old-school pharmacy with a contemporary touch.

Mail-Order Pharmacies:
Do you enjoy online shopping? Then, you will appreciate mail-order pharmacies. They deliver your medications directly to your door, often in 90-day supplies, making life easier and sometimes cheaper, particularly for people with ongoing medication needs. Just make sure you plan ahead so you don't run out.

Hospital Pharmacies:
These are the unsung heroes who manage medications for hospitalized patients. They make certain that everything from pain management to emergency medications is handled perfectly during your stay.

Clinical Pharmacies:
This is where pharmacists step out from behind the counter and work alongside doctors in clinics. They ensure that your drug regimen is as effective as possible, assist your healthcare provider directly in managing chronic conditions, and change or adjust treatments as necessary.

Each pharmacy type offers unique features designed to make your healthcare journey as convenient as possible. Whether you're looking for quick refills, personalized care, or comprehensive support, there's a pharmacy set up to match your healthcare needs, ensuring you receive the care and medications you require in the most convenient way.

1.3: The Journey of a Prescription

Let's break down the process of filling your prescription into clear steps. Whether it's your first time or you need a refresher, this guide will walk you through it. From the moment your doctor prescribes your medications to the time you receive them, you'll be informed every step of the way.

Step 1: Prescription Receipt
When your doctor determines the right medication for you, they will either send it to us directly by e-prescription or hand you a paper prescription to come to us. The advantage of e-prescriptions is their speed; they generally arrive within 15 minutes, allowing us to begin making your medication right away.

Step 2: Check-in at the Pharmacy
When you arrive at the pharmacy, head straight to the "drop-off" counter. This is where you'll provide us with important information like your insurance information and any allergies or sensitivities you may have. It's a

vital step to ensure that we handle your prescription with the utmost care and precision, tailored specifically to your health needs.

Step 3: Prescription Review and Data Entry

A pharmacy team member will then check your prescription for correctness and enter the information into our system. This includes verifying your insurance coverage, checking our stock for your medication, and noting any special handling instructions. Accuracy is essential in this phase to guarantee that your prescription is prepared correctly.

> **Hack:** Don't have insurance or want to save on your medication costs? Make sure to ask us about finding a discount card. We have access to various programs and are experienced at finding the one that offers you the best possible savings on your medications. Additionally, if you've brought any manufacturer coupons, hand them over at this stage to reduce your out-of-pocket expenses.

Step 4: Insurance Authorization

We will contact your insurance company to confirm coverage for your medicine and determine your copay amount. If you're not using insurance, this is when any applicable discounts or coupons will be applied. Should any issues come up, such as the need for prior authorization or if a medication isn't covered, we're here to work with you and your doctor to find a solution.

> **Hack:** Consider consolidating all your prescriptions with us for an added layer of safety and convenience. This streamlines healthcare management and improves our capacity to provide individualized treatment. If we keep a complete record of your prescriptions, we can better prevent potential drug interactions and maximize your overall therapy. It's a proactive move toward preserving your health and making your therapy as effective as possible.

Step 5: Pharmacist Verification

Once the payment details are clear, I'll dive into a thorough review of your prescription and medication history. We're equipped to identify potential medication interactions and duplications, ensuring that your entire regimen works well together.

Step 6: Medication Filling
After we've cleared insurance and safety checks, we'll fill your prescription. This includes accurately preparing, packing, and labeling your medication, as well as providing clear directions for use.

Step 7: Final Pharmacist Check
Before your medication is dispensed, I'll double-check everything for accuracy and correctness, including the medication, dosage, and labeling.

Step 8: Consultation and Pick-Up
When it is time for you to pick up your prescription, we will have a brief but thorough consultation. I'll walk you through how to take your medication properly, warn you about any potential side effects, and answer any questions you might have so that you can feel confident and informed about your treatment.

And there you have it! That's how we get your prescriptions from your doctor's head to your medication cabinet, with a bit of help from your pharmacy team.

> **Hack:** Please keep in mind that our support doesn't end once you've picked up your medication. I'm available for consultations anytime, either in person or over the phone. This can be particularly useful if you're unable to reach your healthcare provider or are unsure about whether to visit urgent care. We're here to provide recommendations and help you decide on the best course of action, including when it's necessary to seek emergency care.

1.4: Refills and Their Rules

Let's explore the world of pharmacy together, shedding light on the refill process, especially when it comes to those complex controlled substances. Understanding this process for your prescriptions is important and straightforward, but it does depend on whether your medication is considered a controlled substance.

Non-controlled Medications:
Refilling non-controlled medications is a flexible process that requires some timing. In general, you can get a refill after using about 80-85% of your current medicine supply. For instance, with a 30-day prescription, you can usually get a refill on day 24. This flexibility allows you to manage your drug levels and get refills as soon as possible, minimizing the risk of treatment interruptions.

Controlled Medications:
Controlled substances face harsher regulations due to their abuse potential. These medications are classified into Schedule II and Schedule III through V, with Schedule II drugs having the strictest regulations.

- **Schedule III through V:** These are medications like alprazolam (Xanax) and tramadol (Ultram). They may be refilled up to five times within six months, with a single pharmacy transfer allowed. Refills for these drugs are usually possible around days 24-28.
- **Schedule II:** This class of medications has the strictest regulations. Schedule II medications, such as hydrocodone/apap (Norco), oxycodone/apap (Percocet), or amphetamine salts (Adderall), cannot be refilled and may only be renewed. Each refill requires a new prescription, which typically cannot be filled sooner than day 28 of a 30-day supply.

> **Hack:** If your prescriber adjusts your medication regimen, such as increasing from 1 to 2 tablets or changing the frequency from 3 to 4 times daily, communicate this with your pharmacist. They may be able to apply a Therapy Change override, allowing you to fill your medication sooner than when the standard turnaround time would be, allowing an early refill for most medications. This approach can also extend to controlled substances but with stricter documentation requirements to ensure compliance with regulations. It's a handy tip for when your treatment plan shifts, ensuring you maintain continuous access to your medication without interruption.

NUANCE: Requesting a refill doesn't automatically mean it's approved; the approval comes from your prescriber. Following up with your doctor's office can speed up this process and ensure your medication is ready when you need it.

Proactive communication with both your healthcare provider and pharmacist is key to staying ahead of potential refill issues. This is especially important for controlled substances, where regulations are stricter. By being proactive, you can ensure you get your medication without interruptions, even when there are regulatory obstacles.

EARLY REFILL REQUESTS:
HANDLING LIFE'S UNEXPECTED TURNS

Life can sometimes throw unexpected situations at us, such as last-minute travel plans or even damaged, lost, or stolen medication. Rest assured that we have solutions in place for these instances. Here are some overrides that your Pharmacist can apply based on your situation. Please remember that these are subject to your insurance plan allowances, as well as having existing refills on your medication.

Vacation Overrides:
This is typically used when extra medication is needed due to travel plans, particularly if you are away for months at a time in another country. Most pharmacies can provide an early refill or an extended amount of medication to cover you during your travel. Some insurance companies do ask for proof of travel plans, so be ready to have that on hand. If not covered, you also have the option to pay out-of-pocket if you have available refills.

Damaged or Lost Medication Override:
If you accidentally drop your medications in a wet sink or can't find them, your pharmacist can use this override to fill an early refill to replace your damaged or lost medication. Just be ready to tell your pharmacist what happened.

Stolen Medication Override:
Similarly, If your medication was stolen, an override may be granted with the necessary proof, such as a police report, depending on your insurance provider's requirements.

REFILL VERSUS RENEWAL:
WHAT'S THE DIFFERENCE?

Understanding the difference between a refill and a renewal is essential for managing your medications effectively. A refill is when you need more of a medication that you have already been prescribed, and you have valid fills remaining based on the original prescription. On the other hand, a renewal requires approval from your healthcare provider to approve additional refills. Both processes are crucial for continuous medication therapy.

> **Hack:** Although not a standard practice, some pharmacists may be able to provide up to a 3-day supply of your medication to bridge the gap, ensuring that your treatment continues without interruption. To do this, you'll need to bring your medication bottle with a valid and complete prescription label to the pharmacy. It's best to go to the pharmacy that originally filled your prescription because they can reprint the label for you. This is particularly useful if you can't bring an empty labeled bottle to the pharmacy. However, if you can't go to the original pharmacy, you can present your labeled bottle to any pharmacy, and they may provide a temporary supply at the pharmacist's discretion. It's important to remember that this only applies to maintenance medications like those for diabetes or blood pressure and not to acute treatments like antibiotics. If a pharmacist is unable to help, don't hesitate to seek another's opinion or visit a different location.

1.5: Prescription Validity Insights

The lifespan of a prescription—how long it remains valid and refillable (meaning it can be renewed for additional doses)— is important for managing medications effectively. This validity varies significantly between non-controlled and controlled substances and depends on federal and state laws, the type of medication, and the choice of each healthcare provider.

Non-Controlled Medications

Non-controlled prescriptions, like those for cholesterol or high blood pressure, are valid for one year from the date they were issued. For instance, if your doctor wrote you a prescription for atorvastatin on January 1, 2023, you should be able to fill it until January 1, 2024, as long as there are refills left. This standard gives patients time to use their refills without having to go to the doctor for the same medication over and over again.

Controlled Medications

Prescriptions for controlled substances are more restricted due to their potential for abuse and dependence.

- **Schedule II** drugs, like oxycodone and Adderall, usually have no refills and are often valid for only 30 days. This means that you need a new order every time you need more medication, which means regular follow-up with your healthcare provider.
- **Schedule III and IV** substances, like testosterone or diazepam, are good for up to six months, and the patient may get up to five refills during that time. For example, if someone is given diazepam on January 1, 2023, the prescription is refillable until June 30, 2023.
- **Schedule V** drugs, like some cough syrups with codeine, are valid for up to one year, similar to non-controlled medications.

State-Specific Variations

It's important to remember that while federal guidelines exist, state laws can modify them to suit local needs better. Some states might have stricter rules, like limiting the use of Schedule II drugs to just seven days for short-term conditions or needing more frequent follow-ups for managing chronic pain. However, these variations are in place to ensure your safety and well-being.

Importance of Regular Consultations

These rules make it even more important to see your doctor regularly to review and renew your medications. This will make sure that you can continue taking your medications safely. Always check your prescriptions to see when they expire, and schedule your doctor visits so that you don't miss any doses, especially if you have a chronic condition.

Knowing how long your prescriptions are good for is important if you want to maintain an uninterrupted medication regimen and follow all safety and legal standards. Equally important is the need for regular consultations with your healthcare provider to review and renew your medications. This ensures that you can continue taking your medications safely and effectively.

1.6: Transfer Process Uncovered

Transferring a prescription from one pharmacy to another is a straightforward process, but it does require some specific steps to ensure that everything is completed accurately and safely. Here's a detailed look at how this process works:

Initiating the Transfer:
The process starts when you, the patient, decide to switch pharmacies for your prescription pick-up. This could be due to various reasons, such as moving to a new area or preferring another pharmacy's services.

Providing Your Details:
Once you've chosen your new pharmacy, you'll need to provide them with some essential information. This includes your full name, date of birth, phone number, and address. It's also important to share relevant health information, such as allergies, and your current insurance details.

Contacting the Current Pharmacy:
After gathering your information, a team member from your newly chosen pharmacy will contact the pharmacy that currently has your prescription. Note: You do not need to contact your previous pharmacy; your new pharmacy team will do all the work of contacting them. Just make sure you share the direct phone number of your previous pharmacy.

Pharmacist-to-Pharmacist Transfer:
Prescription transfers are handled only by pharmacists. They can confirm the transfer details verbally, which is usually done over the phone. A follow-up fax for paperwork may be made following the verbal agreement.

This pharmacist-to-pharmacist interaction guarantees that all information is correctly transmitted and understood.

Timing of the Transfer:
The speed at which your prescription is transferred depends on several factors, including how busy the receiving and transferring pharmacies are at the time of the request. While simple transfers can be done the same day, more complex transfers, such as shifting your whole prescription profile, may take longer—sometimes until the next day or even several days later.

Completion and Confirmation:
Once the transfer is complete, your new pharmacy will have your prescription on file and can begin filling it based on your needs. They'll usually contact you to let you know when your medication is ready for pick-up.

Key Considerations:
Transfers are typically smooth and efficient, but planning can help avoid any lapses in your medication regimen, especially if you're transferring multiple prescriptions or during hectic times for pharmacies. Always ensure that your new pharmacy has all the necessary information, including phone numbers and up-to-date insurance cards, to avoid any delays or billing issues.

TRANSFERRING YOUR PRESCRIPTION:
A CLOSER LOOK

Navigating the complexities of prescription transfers, especially regarding controlled medications, requires a thorough understanding of the process. Let's take a closer look at the process of transferring a prescription.

Non-Controlled Medications:
Transferring prescriptions like Metformin (Glucophage) is typically straightforward. As long as refills exist, pharmacies can transfer your medications from one location to another without issues.

Controlled Substances:
Controlled Medications are not as straightforward. Schedule III through Schedule V medications, such as clonazepam (Klonopin), can be transferred one time with strict record-keeping after they have been filled at least once at the original pharmacy. Schedule II medications, such as hydrocodone/APAP (Norco) or amphetamine salts (Adderall), cannot be transferred. Your healthcare provider would have to issue a new prescription to the pharmacy from which you would like to obtain the medications.

By understanding these processes and utilizing available strategies, such as lost or stolen medication overrides, you can navigate the complexities of medication management more smoothly, ensuring your health care remains continuous and effective.

1.7: Out-of-Stock Solutions

Every now and then, we face the tricky situation where the medication you need isn't immediately available on our shelves. This can be due to supply chain disruptions, sudden spikes in demand, or manufacturing delays. While it's not the most convenient situation, remember that we are in this together. There are several steps we can take, hand in hand, to manage it effectively.

Next-Day Ordering:
First things first—keep calm. If we get our order in before the cutoff time, typically around 5 PM, we can usually get your medication ordered and into your hands by the next business day. Delivery timeframes may vary, but most items ordered are ready for pick-up in the late afternoon, the next business day. Rest assured, we will keep you updated so you know exactly when to stop by.

Speedy Prescription Transfer:
Found a pharmacy with your meds? Great! Provide that pharmacy with our phone number, and they can arrange for your prescription to be transferred. This means they can start prepping your medication immediately

so it's ready when you arrive. Just make sure to provide your contact information so that they can reach you if needed.

TIPS TO STAY AHEAD OF THE GAME

Stay Updated with Text Alerts:
One of the most effective ways to stay informed about medication availability is to sign up for text message alerts. This service makes sure you receive immediate notifications about your prescription status, including availability, ready-for-pick-up alerts, and any out-of-stock notices. Just make sure to read these in detail so you don't confuse whether something is ready to be refilled or whether it is, in fact, ready for pick-up.

Plan Ahead When Possible:
If you are nearing the end of your supply, getting in touch with the pharmacy a few days earlier can make a significant difference. This advance notice gives the pharmacy some wiggle room to manage out-of-stock issues proactively, ensuring your treatment isn't interrupted. By taking this proactive approach, you are taking control of your health and ensuring a seamless treatment process.

> **Hack:** If you can't wait until the next business day, there's a neat trick for those who use big pharmacy chains: quick medication locating. I've seen how these large chains can work wonders for patients. Some pharmacy chains have systems that allow them to check the stock of medications across their other locations, often within a 20-mile radius. Suppose the medication you need isn't available at the pharmacy you visited. In that case, they can quickly find where it is in stock nearby. It's a pretty nifty way to get your hands on your meds without the extra wait.

> **Hack:** Supply concerns may not always be resolved quickly. In such cases, exploring alternative medications with your healthcare provider may be the best course of action. Your pharmacy team can assist by sending a fax to your healthcare provider identifying the supply issue and providing alternative medications that are available to dispense instead.

Keep the Lines Open:
Don't hesitate to discuss your concerns or unique needs with your pharmacy team. They are here to help. Understanding your situation allows them to

prioritize properly and explore every possible option to meet your needs promptly. This reassurance can help build trust and confidence in your healthcare journey.

Remember that an out-of-stock notice does not mean the end of your treatment plan. With proactive planning, utilizing modern pharmacy tools like text alerts, and maintaining open communication with your pharmacy team, you can ensure you continue your treatment seamlessly.

1.8: Backorder Strategies

When you hear "backorder" at the pharmacy, it may appear that your health regimen is about to meet a snag. I'm here with all of my insider expertise to help you manage this situation smoothly.

Unpacking Backorders
A backorder occurs when a medication you need isn't currently available due to delays in manufacturing or supply chain issues. Unlike a quick out-of-stock fix, backorders can be more unpredictable, with sometimes unclear timelines for when the medication will return.

HERE ARE SOME STRATEGIES
FOR HANDLING BACKORDERS

Checking Other Locations:
As with out-of-stock scenarios, your pharmacy team can check the availability of your medication at other pharmacy locations within the same pharmacy chain. If another store has the medication on hand, a transfer can be facilitated to obtain your medication without delay.

Communicating with Your Healthcare Provider:
Your pharmacy team can inform your healthcare provider that your medication is on backorder. Based on your treatment plan, your pharmacist can suggest alternatives, but your healthcare provider does have the final say in approving the alternative or remaining on the current therapy.

Text Alerts:
If you're signed up for text message notifications, you'll receive an update the moment your medication is ready for pick-up; this is especially important if some time has passed and you need reminding that you've been waiting for your medication to get back in stock. This service ensures you're immediately informed.

> **Hack:** Perpetual Ordering—Ask your pharmacy to place your medication on a perpetual order. This means your medication will be automatically ordered and will be processed and filled as soon as it becomes available again, ensuring you're at the front of the line when stock is replenished.

Backorders don't have to derail your treatment. With strategic planning, flexibility, and the proper support from your pharmacy team, you can navigate these challenges effectively.

1.9: Pharmacy's Role in Healthcare

Pharmacies are critical components of the healthcare ecosystem, linking your doctor's recommendations to your daily health routine. Beyond dispensing prescriptions, pharmacists serve as medication safety officers, ensuring that your treatment plan is both safe and effective.

A Critical Checkpoint:
As pharmacists, we are the final checkpoint in your healthcare journey. We meticulously verify that each prescription is correct, look for any drug interactions, and handle any problems that may develop. This attention is equivalent to being a safety officer dedicated to preventing any harm from medication errors.

Partnership with Healthcare Providers:
We collaborate with your healthcare providers to change and manage your prescriptions as needed, ensuring that you receive the most appropriate treatment.

Navigating Insurance and Medication Costs:
It's important to understand that your insurance plan determines the cost of your medications, not the pharmacy. Our role is to process these claims and collect the designated copay. We are also knowledgeable about different insurances and can help troubleshoot with you or your healthcare provider when it comes to insurance rejections.

Empowering Patients:
Our objective is more than just filling prescriptions; we want to provide you with the knowledge and resources you need to make informed healthcare decisions. Our primary goal is to provide you with complete support and guidance.

You don't simply pick up medication at the pharmacy; you also interact with a team dedicated to your health and safety. Remember that every prescription is carefully reviewed by a pharmacist who is committed to your health.

FURTHER READING FOR CHAPTER 1:
EXPLORING THE PHARMACY WORLD

American Pharmacists Association (APhA)
For more information about the roles and responsibilities within the pharmacy team and current pharmacy practices, visit the American Pharmacists Association website. Available at: www.pharmacist.com

Pharmacy Times
Detailed information on different types of pharmacies and their specific functions, as well as insights into the journey of a prescription, can be found at Pharmacy Times. Available at: www.pharmacytimes.com

National Association of Boards of Pharmacy (NABP)
Explore more about prescription transfer processes and how pharmacies handle out-of-stock situations on the National Association of Boards of Pharmacy website. Available at: www.nabp.pharmacy

American Society of Health-System Pharmacists (ASHP)
Comprehensive strategies on managing backorders in pharmacy practice and the broader role of pharmacies in healthcare can be found on the American Society of Health-System Pharmacists website. Available at: www.ashp.org

National Community Pharmacists Association (NCPA)
For insights into pharmacies' overall role in healthcare and how they contribute to patient care, visit the National Community Pharmacists Association, available at www.ncpanet.org.

U.S. National Library of Medicine – MedlinePlus
Provides detailed information on drug information and side effects for a wide range of medications. Available at: medlineplus.gov/druginformation.html

Mayo Clinic
Offers comprehensive health information on the side effects of various medications and tips for managing them. Available at: www.mayoclinic.org.

WebMD – Drugs & Medications A-Z
A resource for learning more about specific drugs and their potential side effects, including management and when to seek medical advice.
Available at: www.webmd.com/drugs/2/index.

Cleveland Clinic – Drug Information
Accessible drug information that includes specific details on managing side effects. Available at: my.clevelandclinic.org/health/drugs.

FDA – Consumer Updates
The U.S. Food and Drug Administration provides updates and articles on drug safety and how to handle side effects effectively.
They are available at www.fda.gov/consumers/consumer-updates.

Harvard Health Publishing – Harvard Medical School
This section features articles on various aspects of medication use, including how to manage side effects and when to consult a healthcare provider. It is available at www.health.harvard.edu/topics/drugs-and-medications.

The Merck Manuals – Online Medical Library
The consumer version offers accessible medical information on medication usage and side effects.
Available at: www.merckmanuals.com/home.

CHAPTER 2:
UNDERSTANDING MEDICATIONS

Welcome to the chapter that will teach you everything you need to know to be a smart medication user. I'm excited to help you figure out what the medication labels mean so you know exactly what, when, and how to take it. The first thing you need to do to take charge of your health is to understand the medications you take. We'll also talk about the important topic of adherence and why taking your medications as prescribed is so important for the success of your treatment. It can be hard to deal with side effects, but we'll learn how to do it together so you can keep your quality of life. We'll also talk about the complicated world of drug interactions, giving you the information you need to avoid problems. Now is the time to give yourself the knowledge and tools you need to make smart choices about your health.

2.1: Decoding Medication Labels

First things first, let's talk about reading medication labels. These are packed with essential information; understanding them is key to managing your health effectively.

Name of the Medication:
Both brand and generic names are important. Knowing both can help you recognize your medication, even if the pharmacy switches between the two.

Dosage:
This tells you how much of the medication is in each pill or liquid form. It's important to ensure you're taking the right amount prescribed by your healthcare provider.

Directions:
Pay close attention here! This section tells you how frequently and how much medication to take. If it reads, "Take one tablet by mouth twice daily," it implies exactly that—not all at once or whenever you remember.

Expiration Date:
Medications do not last forever. Using drugs after their expiration date may mean they are less effective or unsafe.

2.2: Importance of Medication Adherence

Taking your prescription exactly as prescribed is more than just completing a daily duty; it's about getting the most out of your therapy. Missing doses can lead to poor health results, rising healthcare expenses, and a general decline in quality of life. Whether it's for managing chronic conditions like high blood pressure or diabetes, sticking to your prescribed regimen is key to your health's success story.

Let's look at some practical tactics for staying on track, including how to deal with concerns like side effects.

Automatic Refills:
Sign up and let your pharmacy keep track. They'll refill your prescription before it runs out, so you're never without your medications. This also includes proactively reaching out to your healthcare provider for a new prescription when you are out of refills.

Medication Synchronization:
Do you have a handful of prescriptions? Get them to reduce the number of trips you make to the pharmacy, simplifying your routine. It may take a few months for all of your medications to be available on the same day, and even some smaller alignment fills in between, but be patient and let your pharmacy do its thing. Simplicity takes work and patience.

Opt for 90-Day Supplies:
If possible, get a 90-day supply of your meds. Let your pharmacy team know that you prefer to fill 90 days at a time instead of 30 days. This way, they can proactively fill 90 days, including faxing your healthcare provider for 90 days' worth of medication. It's also often cheaper and will reduce your trips to the pharmacy.

Delivery Options:
Many pharmacies now provide delivery, which can range from same-day to 1-2 business days, depending on your preferred timeframe. Larger chains may offer bonuses such as free delivery of certain medications as part of their membership benefits.

> **NUANCE:** It's important to note that there are limitations based on the delivery program offered. Same-day deliveries often require the patient to be present to receive and sign for the delivered medication personally. Also, certain medications, such as controlled substances or refrigerated items, might not be eligible for delivery, or the service might be available only to those with private insurance. Always check the delivery program's specifics or consult the pharmacy offering it for more details. This way, you have the convenience of having your medications delivered right to your door, tailored to fit within the boundaries of the service provided.

Remember, being proactive and involved in your healthcare can lead to better outcomes and a more fulfilling health journey.

2.3: Managing Side Effects

Medications work wonders, but they can also bring some unwanted side effects. Side effects are the body's responses to the chemical changes that medications cause. Navigating the twists and turns of medication side effects can be smoother with some know-how. I'm here to guide you through managing those side effects so you can focus on feeling better without unnecessary discomfort.

Nausea:
Medications like antibiotics and chemotherapy can upset your stomach.

> **Solution:** Ginger tea or ginger candies can be natural remedies for nausea. Additionally, try to take these medications with a light meal or snack unless your healthcare provider advises otherwise.

Dizziness:
Blood pressure medications, anti-seizure drugs, and even some antidepressants might leave you feeling lightheaded.

> **Solution:** Get up slowly from sitting or lying positions and stay hydrated. If the dizziness doesn't go away or improve, speak with your doctor, as your medication may need to be adjusted.

Headaches:
Various medications, including those for erectile dysfunction, such as sildenafil (Viagra), and certain weight loss drugs, such as phentermine, may cause headaches as a side effect.

> **Solution:** Stay hydrated. Taking a mild OTC pain treatment as recommended by your pharmacist and avoiding stressors such as loud noises or bright lights will help.

Constipation:
Iron supplements, opiates, and certain high-blood pressure medications are known to slow down the digestive system.

> **Solution:** Increase your fiber intake by eating more fruits, vegetables, and whole grains, and if your doctor agrees, use a light, over-the-counter stool softener.

Insomnia:

Stimulants used for ADHD, corticosteroids, and some antidepressants can interfere with sleep.

> **Solution:** Limit your caffeine intake during the day, stick to a normal bedtime routine, and talk to your doctor about taking your prescription in the morning.

TIPS FOR MANAGING SIDE EFFECTS

Hydration is Key:
Increased water intake can help with a variety of adverse effects, including dry mouth and lightheadedness.

Dietary Adjustments:
Some side effects are lessened by food, so learn whether to take your medication with a meal or on an empty stomach.

The addition of fiber to the diet can aid with constipation while limiting caffeine intake can help with sleep.

Custom Timing:
For meds that cause drowsiness, taking them before bedtime can help. On the other hand, morning administration is key for those that might keep you awake.

Temperature Tricks:
For injections that cause irritation, applying a cold pack before and a warm compress after can reduce discomfort.

Stay Informed:
Know the potential side effects of your medications. The more you know, the better prepared you will be to deal with them. It's also vital to know which side effects are more than nuisances. Severe reactions require immediate medical attention. Contact your pharmacist or healthcare provider if you're experiencing anything alarming.

Write it down:
Documenting when you take your medications and any side effects you encounter can be extremely beneficial in controlling and reporting these issues with your healthcare provider

Open Communication:
If you are experiencing any adverse effects, contact your pharmacist or healthcare practitioner. There may be alternatives or tactics you can use to reduce your discomfort.

The FDA and MedlinePlus are excellent resources for learning more about managing medication side effects. Remember that while side effects are a normal part of the treatment process, they should not outweigh the advantages. With the right knowledge and tactics, you can manage them effectively and keep your focus on your health and recovery.

2.4: Medication Interactions Simplified

When it comes to managing medication interactions, having a central location for all of your prescriptions is essential. This approach enables your pharmacist to conduct a comprehensive review of potential drug interactions, ensuring that your treatment plan is both safe and effective. It's not just prescription medications that need to be considered; over-the-counter (OTC) drugs, herbal supplements, and natural remedies also play a huge role in this complex web of interactions. Let's look at some examples of how combining certain medications can sometimes do more harm than good, particularly when dealing with common health conditions.

Diabetes Medications (ex., metformin)
Metformin is often prescribed for managing diabetes. However, when paired with contrast dye, which is used in certain radiology procedures, there is an increased risk of developing lactic acidosis, a severe buildup of lactic acid in the body. To avoid this risk, inform your healthcare provider about your Metformin use before undergoing such procedures.

Heartburn Medications (ex., omeprazole)
Because they can lower stomach acidity, proton pump inhibitors (PPIs) such as Omeprazole can affect the absorption of vital nutrients and other drugs. They have the potential to damage bones over time by affecting calcium absorption. They can also interfere with the effectiveness of certain antifungal and antiviral drugs, requiring careful monitoring and, in some cases, dosage modifications.

Thyroid Medications (ex., levothyroxine)
These require careful timing with your meals and other medications. Calcium supplements, iron tablets, and even some multivitamins can affect the absorption of thyroid medications, requiring a gap of at least four hours between these and your thyroid medication.

Blood thinners (ex.clopidogrel)
Clopidogrel (Plavix) is prescribed to prevent blood clots, but it must be used with caution when combined with over-the-counter NSAIDs like ibuprofen. When taken together, NSAIDs can affect how well clopidogrel works, potentially resulting in severe bleeding or clotting problems. Before adding or changing medications, it's important to consult with your healthcare provider and stay on top of regular blood tests.

High Blood Pressure Medications (ex., amlodipine)
Patients on high blood pressure medications should be careful when using over-the-counter decongestants such as pseudoephedrine (Sudafed) and phenylephrine, which are present in many cold and flu treatments. Decongestants can raise blood pressure and heart rate, reversing the benefits of blood pressure medications such as amlodipine and posing risks to patients with heart conditions.

Asthma or COPD Medications (ex., Albuterol)
For patients suffering from asthma or COPD, combining different inhalers without sufficient advice can result in excessive doses of similar drugs. For example, using albuterol (Proair) with other beta-agonists, such as salmeterol, without coordination increases the risk of side effects such as jitteriness and heart palpitations and may even worsen breathing issues.

Cholesterol-lowering Medications (ex., Simvastatin)
Lastly, patients taking statins such as simvastatin should be aware of interactions with grapefruit juice. Grapefruit juice can raise the medication's blood levels, increasing the likelihood of side effects such as muscle pain or weakness, both of which indicate muscle breakdown. This seemingly simple dietary choice can affect how safe and effective these medications are.

Understanding your medications doesn't have to be a chore. Consider it an important step in taking control of your health. Remember, my door (or pharmacy counter) is always open for you to ask questions, express concerns, or chat about the newest in health and wellness. Together, we'll make sure you're informed, confident, and ready to face your medication regimen head-on. Here's to your health!

FURTHER READING FOR CHAPTER 2:
UNDERSTANDING MEDICATIONS

Institute for Safe Medication Practices (ISMP)
Learn about best practices for safe medication use, including how to effectively manage medication interactions, from the Institute for Safe Medication Practices. Available at: www.ismp.org.

Centers for Disease Control and Prevention (CDC) – Medication Safety Program
This website provides information on safe medication use, preventing medication errors, and managing side effects.
It is available at www.cdc.gov/medicationsafety/index.html.

U.S. Food and Drug Administration (FDA) – Drug Information
Offers comprehensive resources on drug interactions, side effects, drug safety communications, and consumer updates. Available at: www.fda.gov/drugs.

National Institutes of Health (NIH) – MedlinePlus
This is a reliable, up-to-date drug information resource, including a medical encyclopedia and information on over-the-counter and prescription drugs.
It is available at: medlineplus.gov/druginformation.html.

Mayo Clinic – Drugs and Supplements
It offers user-friendly information on medications, including detailed descriptions of drug interactions and side effects.
It is available at www.mayoclinic.org/drugs-supplements.

National Center for Complementary and Integrative Health (NCCIH)
Offers evidence-based information on various natural remedies and their effects, including herbs and supplements for different health conditions.
Available at: www.nccih.nih.gov.

WebMD – Medication Management
Provides practical tips on managing medications, understanding potential side effects, and interactions between drugs.
Available at: www.webmd.com/drugs/2/drug-conditions

CHAPTER 3:

MEDICATION MANAGEMENT MASTERY

This is where I'll be giving you some insider tips on how to handle your medications better, so let's get down to business. First, we'll go over the basics of how to take your medications so that you can be sure you're getting the most out of them. Taking on complicated routines? I know some simple tricks that will make it easy for you to stay on track. Did you forget to take your medications? Don't worry, I'll show you what to do next. We will also talk about some easy ways to make taking pills a breeze if you are having trouble with it. I'll also cover side effects and give you tips on how to handle them like a pro. We'll clear up any misunderstanding about when medications have expired so you know when to throw away old pills. Let's make it easy to take our medications together!

3.1: Administering Medications Correctly

The effectiveness of your treatment often hinges not just on what medication you take but also on how you take it. From topical creams to complex injectables, the method of administration has a huge impact on how well the medication works and your experience. Let's dive into the proper usage of various medication forms, ensuring that you are completely prepared to manage your or a loved one's healthcare needs efficiently.

Creams and Ointments

These are applied to the skin to treat conditions like eczema or arthritis. For example, hydrocortisone cream reduces inflammation and itching. Prior to use, make sure the skin is clean and dry. Apply a thin layer to the area that's affected and gently massage until absorbed. Avoid using a bandage unless advised by your healthcare provider. Putting a bandage over topical medications can cause more medication to be absorbed.

Injectables

Medications like insulin for diabetes or vitamin B12 shots are administered via injection. For insulin, it's crucial to rotate injection sites to prevent tissue damage. Repeated injections at the same site can lead to hard lumps or fatty deposits. Always use a new needle and make sure the injection site is clean by wiping it with an alcohol pad first. For subcutaneous injections, pinch the skin slightly; relax the muscle as much as possible for intramuscular injections.

Patches

Transdermal patches, like those used for pain relief (e.g., fentanyl patches) or smoking cessation (nicotine patches), provide a steady release of medication through the skin. Apply the patch to a clean, dry, hairless part of the skin, typically the upper torso or upper arm. Avoid areas with cuts or irritation. Press down for about 30 seconds to make sure the patch sticks well. Note the application time and date since most patches need regular changing. Check the package for specific manufacturer instructions on how to apply since some may have specific needs or should not be used at all.

Eye Drops

Proper administration is key. These are typically used for conditions like glaucoma or dry eyes. Tilt your head back, pull down your lower eyelid to form a "pocket," and drop the medication into it without touching the tip of the dropper to your eye. Blink slowly a few times and gently press on the inner corner to keep the drop from draining away. Don't use eye drops past their expiration date or if you notice changes in the color or clarity of the drops.

Ear Drops

Ear drops are typically used for ear infections or to soften earwax. Warm the bottle in your hands for a few minutes before use. Lie down with the affected ear pointing up. Pull the earlobe up and back to straighten the ear canal, then use the drops. Stay in this position for a few minutes to let the medication get fully absorbed deep into the ear. Don't use ear drops if you think there is damage to the eardrum unless instructed by your healthcare provider.

Nasal Sprays

These are often used for allergies or congestion. Blow your nose gently before use. Tilt your head slightly forward, insert the tip of the spray into one nostril, and press while breathing in. To allow the medication to take effect, avoid blowing your nose right away.

TIPS FOR MEDICATION ADMINISTRATION

In-depth Demonstrations:
If you have never used a medication form before, ask your pharmacist for a demonstration. They can offer tips and advice suited to your particular medication.

Use of Administering Aids:
For difficult-to-use forms, like eye drops, consider devices such as Eye Drop Helpers, which are meant to help with the application. Ask your pharmacist about these aids.

Consistency in Technique:
Consistency is key, especially with injectables and drops. Create a routine that includes reviewing the clarity and expiration dates before each usage.

Follow-up:
Make follow-up appointments with your healthcare provider to discuss your medication experience, any side effects, and whether the treatment is functioning as intended.

Understanding the nuances of each medication form and following best practices ensures you get the most out of your treatments. If you have any issues or need extra information about your prescription regimen, always contact your healthcare team.

3.2: Managing Complex Regimens

Managing multiple medications can sometimes feel overwhelming, especially in forms like eye drops, ear drops, creams, or inhalers. Knowing which medication to use first and how long to wait between doses can affect the effectiveness of the medications. Let's explore key considerations and tips to make this process smoother and maximize each medication's efficiency.

Eye Drops

When using multiple eye drops, allow at least 5 to 10 minutes between each drop. This keeps the second drop from washing out the first, giving both drugs enough time to be absorbed. If you're using both an eye drop and an eye ointment, apply the drops first and the ointment last since applying the ointment first can create a barrier, keeping the eye drops from being absorbed well.

> **Example:** If you're using a lubricating drop and a glaucoma drop, apply the glaucoma drop first, wait for about 5-10 minutes, then follow with the lubricating drop.

Ear Drops

If you need to use multiple ear drops, you should space them apart, just like you would with eye drops. A good rule of thumb is to provide at least 5 minutes between different types.

> **Example:** If you're treating an ear infection with both an antibiotic drop and a steroid drop, start with the antibiotic, wait, and then use the steroid drop.

Topical Creams and Ointments

Multiple creams, like eye and ear drops, must be spaced apart when used or applied to the same location. Apply the lighter consistency first and let it seep into your skin before applying the thicker cream.

> **Example:** For skin conditions that need both a medicated cream and a moisturizing ointment, apply the medicated cream first, let it absorb, and then follow with the ointment. Some topical medications may interact with each other and need specific timing, so confirm with your healthcare provider or pharmacist first.

Injectables: Single Dose vs. Multi-Dose

Understanding whether your injectable medication is a single dose or multi-dose can affect how you plan your administration. Single-dose vials are intended for one-time use only, even if they contain more medication than is required for a single dose. Multi-dose vials are designed for multiple uses, with specific storage instructions and expiration dates after opening. They may have enough for two months but expire one month after opening, so paying attention to expiration dates is critical. Always use alcohol wipes to clean the vial's top before each dose.

> **Example:** Insulin is often in multi-dose vials, allowing you to use the same vial multiple times. Certain injectable testosterones are in single-dose vials to be used once and discarded, even if extra is left for another use.

Inhalers

When using multiple inhalers, such as albuterol, a bronchodilator, and fluticasone, a corticosteroid, the order of administration makes a big difference. First, use the bronchodilator inhaler to open your airways, followed by the corticosteroid inhaler about 5 minutes later. This lets the steroid get deeper into the lungs. It's also important to use proper inhaler technique and to regularly clean the inhaler to make sure it continues to work well and to keep good hygiene.

Example: To manage asthma, use an albuterol inhaler (bronchodilator) before a fluticasone inhaler (corticosteroid).

HERE ARE SOME TIPS TO HELP YOU
MANAGE THESE MORE COMPLEX REGIMENS

Create a Medication Schedule:
Write down when and in what order you should take your prescriptions or use a digital organizer to keep track of them.

Label Everything:
Use stickers or markers to label your pills with the time they should be taken and in what order, especially if you have a complicated regimen.

Practice Proper Technique:
Use the correct technique for each medication form. If you need more clarification, your pharmacist can demonstrate the proper method.

Understanding the significance of the order and timing of medication administration, particularly when administering multiple medications, can help ensure that each treatment is as effective as possible.

3.3: Dealing with Missed Doses

Navigating missed doses can be a difficult aspect of health management, especially when juggling treatments for disorders such as high cholesterol, diabetes, high blood pressure, and asthma or while taking antidepressants and birth control pills. Here's a friendly guide to help you stay on track.

Birth Control Pills
Missed One Pill: Take it as soon as you remember, then continue with your next dose at the regular time (even if it means taking two pills in one day). Your protection against pregnancy should remain effective.

Missed Two or More: Take the most recent missed pill right away and toss any previously missed ones. Use backup contraception (such as condoms) for the next seven days while keeping your regular schedule.

High Cholesterol (Statins like Atorvastatin)
If it has been less than 12 hours since your missed dose, take it as soon as you remember. If it has been more than 12 hours, don't take the missing dose and continue with your regular dosage. Don't double-up doses. This keeps beneficial levels while keeping you from taking too much.

Diabetes (Oral Medications like Metformin)
If you remember missing a dose the same day, take it with your next meal. If you remember it the next day, skip it and take your next dose as scheduled. Never take a double dose. This will help keep your blood sugar levels steady without lowering them too much.

High Blood Pressure (ACE Inhibitors like Lisinopril)
If you remember within 12 hours of missing a dosage, take it as soon as you remember. If it's nearing the time of your next dose, skip it. Maintaining a steady amount in your blood is critical, but don't double up to catch up. This keeps your blood pressure from dropping too much.

Asthma (Inhalers like Albuterol)
If you forget a dose, take it as soon as you remember. Asthma medication dosing is based on the frequency and severity of symptoms, so missing a dose is not as important as taking your dose and addressing your symptoms. Inhalers can usually be used regularly or whenever it's needed.

Antidepressants (SSRIs like Sertraline)
If it is less than half the time until your next dose, take it as soon as you remember. If it has been more than half, skip it and take the next dose at your usual time. Do not double up. Sudden changes in your doses can affect your mood or cause side effects. Taking antidepressants regularly is important to avoid withdrawal signs and mood swings.

GENERAL TIPS
FOR HANDLING MISSED DOSES

Set Alarms:
Use alarms on your phone or pill reminder applications to stay on track.

Understand Your Medication:
Understanding the purpose and effects of your medication can help you stay on your medication regimen.

90-Day Prescriptions:
Consider requesting a 90-day supply from your healthcare provider for long-term medications that you regularly take, such as those for chronic diseases like diabetes. It's more convenient and can help you stay on top of taking your medications timely.

When in Doubt:
Always contact your healthcare provider or pharmacist if you need help with a missed dosage of your specific medication, especially for medical conditions not covered here. We are your health allies, committed to ensuring that your treatment is effective and that your journey to wellness goes smoothly.

3.4: Techniques for Pill Swallowing

Trouble swallowing pills shouldn't stand in the way of your health. If you have difficulty swallowing pills, know that you are not alone, and it shouldn't keep you from taking your medications. There are several tricks and alternative methods to make swallowing pills easier, ensuring you can still receive the benefits of your treatments without the stress. Let's look at some practical strategies and tricks for overcoming this common issue.

Tablets:
First and foremost, it's important to know that not all drugs are created equal. Some tablets have scores (lines) in the middle, allowing them to be cut in half safely. This can make swallowing easier. However, always

consult with your pharmacist before splitting any medications since not all tablets can be cut in half safely.

Capsules:

These offer their own set of options. They can sometimes be opened, and the contents sprinkled on a small amount of food (such as applesauce or yogurt). However, not all capsules are intended to be opened. It's important to get the green light from your healthcare provider or pharmacist first.

> **NUANCE:** ER (extended-release) and CR (controlled-release) drugs are specifically designed to release the medication slowly. Crushing, chewing, or breaking them can release all of the medication at once, which can lead to side effects or decreased effectiveness. Always take these pills whole. Some capsules can be opened and sprinkled even though they are ER or CR; however, always check with your healthcare provider or pharmacist to see if your capsule is one of these exceptions.

Now, let's talk about some techniques that can help:

The Pop Bottle Method:

This method works best with tablets. Fill a flexible plastic bottle with water, place the tablet on your tongue, then close your lips around the bottle opening and take a drink, swallowing the water and tablet together. The water and swallowing action can help the tablet go down smoothly.

The Lean Forward Method:

This is especially useful for capsules. Place the capsule on top of your tongue and take a sip of water, but do not swallow immediately. Instead, tilt your head forward, chin to chest. In this position, the capsule will float to the back of your mouth, making it simpler to swallow while drinking water.

These hacks and methods are designed to ease the pill-swallowing process. Still, the most important advice is to communicate with your healthcare provider or pharmacist. We're here to help you find the best solution, whether it's exploring medication alternatives, adjusting your technique, or providing more personalized tips.

3.5: Mitigating Side Effects

It's important to know that side effects are essentially your body's way of adjusting to the new medication or substance. Whether you're taking medications for high blood pressure, diabetes, or asthma, side effects can range from drowsiness to stomach problems. I'm here to provide some tips on how to deal with these side effects and make your journey to health as comfortable as possible.

Here are some ways to manage side effects from common medications taken for chronic health conditions.

High Blood Pressure Medications (ex., Lisinopril)
People taking blood pressure medications such as Lisinopril may experience a dry cough. Drinking water and staying hydrated helps. If it gets too bothersome, it might be time to switch to an alternative therapy. Talk to your healthcare provider or pharmacist about your options.

Diabetes Medications (ex., Metformin)
Managing side effects from diabetic medications takes patience, knowledge, and, in some cases, lifestyle changes. Metformin, a common diabetes medication, can cause pain in the stomach and intestines, which can usually be helped by taking the medication with a meal to buffer its effects. If taking it with meals doesn't help, asking your healthcare provider for the extended-release version of Metformin may provide relief while maintaining the effectiveness of the medication. Adding regular exercise and being hydrated can also help reduce potential side effects and increase the effectiveness of your diabetes treatment.

Asthma Inhalers (ex., Albuterol)
Those using asthma inhalers such as Albuterol may develop jitteriness, which often decreases with regular use. To reduce this side effect, incorporating relaxation techniques such as yoga, deep breathing exercises, and progressive muscular relaxation can help. Staying hydrated and avoiding

caffeine and other stimulants can also help to reduce jitteriness. If these symptoms persist or worsen, talk with a healthcare provider to possibly adjust the medication or explore other treatment options.

Statins (ex., Atorvastatin for High Cholesterol)
Statins, used for managing high cholesterol, might lead to muscle aches. Regular, moderate exercise and staying hydrated can help reduce these symptoms. However, severe muscle aches mean something more severe, and your medication might need to be adjusted or replaced with an alternative. Talk with your healthcare provider if you have constant or severe muscle aches without anything causing them, such as excessive exercise, especially if you also have dark urine or feel tired.

Oral Contraceptives (Birth Control Pills)
Consistency is essential for people taking oral contraceptives, especially for those who are experiencing mood swings or nausea. Taking your medication at the same time every day can help regulate hormone levels, and taking it with food or at bedtime reduces nausea and stomach aches.

Mood Stabilizers (ex., Sertraline)
Common side effects range from insomnia and sexual dysfunction with SSRIs like sertraline (Zoloft), nausea and elevated blood pressure with SNRIs like duloxetine (Cymbalta), and dry mouth and constipation with TCAs like amitriptyline (Elavil). Managing these effects can be accomplished by adjusting medication timing. Taking SSRIs in the morning or taking TCAs with food would help. Simple lifestyle changes, such as staying hydrated or eating sugar-free candy, can help with dry mouth. Communicate concerns and side effects with your healthcare provider or pharmacist so they can help you manage your side effects or offer alternative medications or dosage adjustments. Before making changes to your medications, you should always talk to a healthcare provider first.

Side effects should not prevent you from achieving your health goals. Most can be properly managed with the right strategies and a bit of patience.

3.6: Risk of Expired Medications

Important Disclaimer: I, the author, do not endorse or recommend using expired medications. Always consult a healthcare professional, such as a pharmacist or doctor, before making decisions about your medication.

When it comes to using medications past their expiration dates, it's always a bit of a tightrope walk. While some meds might be okay to use for a short time after their expiration date, others can become less effective or even unsafe. Let's break it down:

MEDICATIONS THAT ARE GENERALLY **OKAY TO USE** PAST THEIR EXPIRATION (BUT STILL, USE WITH CAUTION)

Over-the-Counter Pain Relievers
Medications like aspirin, acetaminophen (Tylenol), ibuprofen (Advil), and naproxen (Aleve) can retain most of their efficacy after their expiration date if stored in optimal storage conditions. However, their effectiveness reduces over time, so they won't be providing effective pain relief if they are significantly expired.

Antihistamines (Claritin, Zyrtec, Benadryl):
Used for allergy relief, loratadine (Claritin), cetirizine (Zyrtec), and diphenhydramine (Benadryl) may still be effective after their expiration dates. However, like pain medications, how well they work gradually declines after their expiration dates and may not provide effective allergy relief.

Stomach Acid Medications:
Proton pump inhibitors (PPIs) like Omeprazole and H2 blockers such as famotidine (Pepcid) may continue to work after their expiration date, especially if stored in ideal storage conditions, such as away from moisture and heat.

MEDICATIONS THAT NEED TO BE *USED WITH CAUTION* (MUST CONSULT WITH PHARMACIST OR HEALTHCARE PROVIDER)

Prescription Medications:
The FDA's Shelf Life Extension Program (SLEP) has found that certain medications such as amlodipine and lisinopril for high blood pressure, atorvastatin and simvastatin for high cholesterol, and metformin for diabetes, and levothyroxine for thyroid therapy retain their efficacy after their expiration dates. This program studies and highlights some drugs that continue to work after their labeled expiration date. However, this extended efficacy only applies to medications stored in ideal conditions, which is not typically achieved in home environments. Medications stored at home are exposed to variable temperatures, humidity, and light, all of which can affect their stability and potency.

Tablet Form of Medications
Tablets generally have a longer shelf life compared to liquids, suspensions, or solutions. Antibiotic tablets such as amoxicillin and ciprofloxacin can remain stable and effective for some time beyond their expiration dates, whereas their liquid counterparts are unsafe to use.

MEDICATIONS THAT ARE *UNSAFE TO USE* PAST THEIR EXPIRATION DATES

Insulin:
Insulins, used to control blood sugar in diabetes, can lose their blood-glucose-lowering effects after the expiration date. For safety and efficacy, they must be used within their specified shelf life.

Nitroglycerin:
Typically used for angina, it is highly sensitive to degradation. It can lose its effectiveness quickly once the bottle is opened, even more so when it is past its expiration date. Sublingual tablets are particularly sensitive once the bottle is opened. It's recommended that they be replaced every six months.

Antibiotics:

Particularly, liquid antibiotics can degrade chemically and physically after their expiration date, which is usually a few days after they are reconstituted or mixed. This means they may fail to treat infections, causing antibiotic resistance and even becoming harmful. Antibiotics vary in how stable they are after being mixed, make sure to read and follow storage instructions and get rid of any leftover medication after the time period provided on the labeling or instructions.

Eye Drops:

Using eye drops, particularly the preservative-free kind, is unsafe and can even cause eye infections. It's important not to use eye drops that have passed their expiration date because they might not work as well or could get contaminated.

EpiPens and Other Emergency Medications:

EpiPens contain epinephrine, which is critical for treating severe allergic reactions. However, their potency diminishes after the expiration date, making them unreliable in emergency situations. Reliability in life-threatening situations is too important to compromise.

> **Hack:** Examine your medicine cabinet on a regular basis and remove any expired medications. Use pharmacy take-back programs to ensure safe and environmentally friendly disposal. This approach keeps your medication regimen functional and protects your health by avoiding the use of possibly ineffective or harmful expired prescriptions.

It's important to consult with a healthcare professional, such as a pharmacist, before using any medication after its expiration date. The FDA and healthcare professionals warn against using outdated medications because they pose a risk to your health. Always prioritize safety, and when in doubt, don't use it.

Wrapping it all up...

Managing your prescriptions doesn't have to be a complex puzzle. With these practical tips and your pharmacist as a resource, you can be confident that your drug regimen is not only tailored to your needs but is also safe and effective.

FURTHER READING FOR CHAPTER 3:
MEDICATION MANAGEMENT MASTERY

American Pharmacists Association (APhA)
Explore guidance on administering medications correctly and managing complex medication regimens from the American Pharmacists Association.
Available at: www.pharmacist.com.

Institute for Safe Medication Practices (ISMP)
For expert advice on dealing with missed doses and techniques for pill swallowing, check out resources available at the Institute for Safe Medication Practices.
Available at: www.ismp.org

Mayo Clinic
Learn about mitigating side effects and ensuring safe medication use from the Mayo Clinic's comprehensive patient care resources.
Available at: www.mayoclinic.org

U.S. Food and Drug Administration (FDA)
Understand the risks associated with expired medications and the importance of proper medication disposal from the U.S. Food and Drug Administration.
Available at: www.fda.gov.

Centers for Disease Control and Prevention (CDC) – Injection Safety
Offers comprehensive information on safe injection practices to prevent infections.
Available at: www.cdc.gov/injectionsafety/patients/index.html.

National Institutes of Health (NIH) – MedlinePlus – How to Take Medicines
Provides patients with education on how to take medicines correctly, including the use of patches, eye drops, and more.
Available at: medlineplus.gov/howtotakemedicines.html

The Merck Manuals – Online Medical Library
The consumer version offers detailed explanations on how medications should be administered, emphasizing safety and effectiveness.
Available at: www.merckmanuals.com/home.

CHAPTER 4:
INSURANCE NAVIGATION

Health insurance can be like trying to read an old script: it's hard to find your way around, and it can be a puzzle. Don't worry, though! We're about to go on a trip to defeat this beast together. I'll teach you the basics of health insurance and help you figure out what the terms mean for you. I'll help you get the medications you need and tackle the complicated process of prior authorizations. You'll learn how to use insurance formularies wisely to save not only dollars but maybe even hundreds! We'll also talk about primary and secondary insurance to make sure you get the most out of your coverage while keeping costs as low as possible. And if you need to argue a decision, I'll teach you how to do it right so you can stand up for your rights. I'll also cover how to work with your healthcare team to get the most out of your coverage and even how to get medication refunds. It's time to learn how to use your insurance wisely and turn your frustration into control!

4.1: Health Insurance Basics

Navigating the realm of health insurance is essential for managing both your health and financial well-being. Health insurance protects against the high costs of healthcare services and medications. Here are some important terms and concepts to get started.

KEY INSURANCE
TERMS EXPLAINED

Deductibles:
This is the amount you must spend for healthcare services, which can be charged through your prescriptions or doctor's office visits before your insurance policy starts to contribute. For example, if your deductible is $1,000, you are responsible for the first $1,000 in healthcare costs each year.

Co-pays:
These are predetermined fees that you pay for specific medical services or prescription pick-ups under your health insurance plan. For example, a co-pay could be $25 for a doctor's office visit or $15 for a medication refill.

Co-insurance:
After you've reached your deductible, co-insurance is the percentage of the cost of a service that you pay. For example, if you have a 20% co-insurance rate and the service costs $200, you will pay $40 while insurance covers the remaining $160.

Practical Example: Consider this scenario: your prescription drug costs $200, and you've already reached your annual deductible. If your co-insurance rate is 20%, you will pay $40 out of cash for that medication, while your insurance will cover the rest, $160. However, if your plan has a co-pay of $15 for your medications, you will only pay that amount, regardless of the overall cost.

Hack: Always keep a current copy of your formulary handy. It can change; what was covered last year or during previous years might not be this year. You often have the option to choose your insurance based on coverage of your current medications. Usually, your insurance plan has a member helpline to assist you in selecting the best plan for you.

Formularies:
A formulary is a comprehensive list of medications covered by your insurance plan, which often includes both generic and brand-name drugs. Medications on this list are typically less expensive, making it beneficial to choose these options when possible.

4.2: Prior Authorizations Explained

When you're ready to start a new medication but encounter a roadblock called prior authorization, it might feel like a major inconvenience. However, understanding why it's necessary can simplify the process and help guide you through your next steps.

The Reason Behind It:
Prior authorizations are a process that insurance companies use to ensure that the prescribed medication is both necessary for your treatment and is a cost-effective option.

Steps You Can Take:
Once the pharmacy informs you that your medication requires prior authorization, call your healthcare provider and let them know that a prior authorization is needed for the medication they just prescribed. This will significantly speed up the process. Your healthcare provider is required to provide your insurance with additional details about your medication so that it can be covered. Proactively following up with both your healthcare provider and your insurance company can expedite the approval process.

> **Hack:** Remember that prior authorizations are all about insurance coverage. If waiting for approval is not an option or you're open to covering the cost independently, let your pharmacist know that you want to proceed without insurance. This is your cue to ask about potential savings through discount cards or manufacturer coupons. You can also ask your pharmacist to recommend an alternative medication that is covered by your insurance, after which you can request a new prescription from your doctor's office.

A PRO Tip: Documenting how your medical condition affects your daily life will help your doctor make a stronger argument to your insurance company about why this specific medication is necessary for you.

4.3: Insurance Formularies and Cost Savings

Diving into insurance formularies may not sound like an exciting adventure, but it's one worth taking for anyone looking to save money on medications. An insurance formulary is essentially a list of medications that your insurance plan prefers and covers. These medications are chosen based on their efficacy, safety, and cost-effectiveness. Formularies are often divided into tiers. As we go up in tier, the out-of-pocket cost increases for you, the patient.

Tier 1: Generic Medications
These are the most affordable medications on an insurance plan. They are typically generic equivalents of brand-name prescriptions and contain the same active ingredients, strength, and dosage forms as the brand-name products but are significantly less expensive.

Tier 2: Preferred Brand-Name Medications
These are brand-name medications that the insurance plan pays for at a greater cost than generics but less than non-preferred drugs. They are often chosen for their affordability and effectiveness.

Tier 3: Non-Preferred Brand-Name Medications
This tier covers brand-name medications that are not recommended due to the availability of less expensive generic or preferred brand-name alternatives. These drugs require higher copays or coinsurance. Drugs in this tier could include newer, more expensive medications that don't have generics yet.

Tier 4: Specialty Medications
These are expensive prescription medications often used to treat complex, chronic diseases such as cancer, multiple sclerosis, and rheumatoid arthritis. They may require special handling, administration, or monitoring.

Due to their advanced technology or treatment capabilities, specialty medications are frequently the most expensive for patients out-of-pocket.

> **Hack:** Determine which tier your drug fits into. If it is higher than Tier 1, ask your pharmacist or doctor to see if a generic or lower-tier alternative could work for you.

Understanding your insurance's medication tiers can help you and your healthcare provider make more informed treatment decisions and better manage your medication costs.

HOW TO USE FORMULARIES FOR SAVINGS

Review Your Plan's Formulary:
Start by getting the most recent version of your insurance's formulary. This is normally available on the insurer's website or by contacting customer service.

Discuss Alternatives with Your Healthcare Provider:
If you are prescribed a medication that is high on the tier list (and thus more expensive), discuss possible lower-tier alternatives with your doctor. There could be a generic or another brand-name prescription that is just as effective but less expensive.

Check for Updates:
Formularies are reviewed and can change on a yearly basis. Thus, a medication that was covered at a reduced cost one year may move to a higher tier the following year. Stay up to date on any changes to avoid unexpected costs.

Appeal Decisions:
If you are taking a medication that is not on the formulary or has been placed in a higher-cost tier, you and your doctor can file an appeal with your insurance company. Providing documentation explaining why a specific medication is important for your health may lead to coverage exceptions.

Ask Your Pharmacist for Help:
Your pharmacist is an excellent source of information about your insurance formulary. They can often propose alternatives and assist you in navigating the nuances of your plan.

By using your insurance formulary wisely, you can make more informed decisions about your medications, potentially saving you on costs over time. Remember that being proactive about your prescription costs is not just smart; it is essential in managing your overall healthcare expenses.

4.4: Understanding Primary vs. Secondary Insurance

Navigating your coverage when you have multiple health insurance plans can feel like a jigsaw puzzle. But don't worry—I'm here to make things easier. Understanding the roles of primary and secondary insurance cannot only help you save time but also maximize your benefits.

PRIMARY VS. SECONDARY INSURANCE EXPLAINED

Primary Insurance:
This insurance plan pays first when you have a healthcare expense. It covers its portion of the costs, based on your plan's benefits, before any other insurance is considered. If you are employed and have insurance through your employer, this is usually your primary insurance.

Hack: If your insurer declines a claim because it believes another insurer should cover it, contact both insurers to coordinate the benefits. Your insurers need to know if they are the primary or secondary. Typically, insurance from your job is the primary insurance, and your spouse's coverage would be your secondary. If you have two jobs, the primary is the job that you work the most hours at. This step is important to avoid out-of-pocket expenses.

Secondary insurance:
This kicks in after your primary insurer has paid its portion, covering any additional fees or co-pays that the primary did not cover. Consider it a safety net that helps lower your out-of-pocket costs.

Coordination of Benefits (COB):
This is the process by which your insurers communicate to determine who pays first (primary) and who pays later (secondary). The goal is to avoid duplicate payments or overinsurance. If you are insured by your spouse's and your employer's policies, one will be deemed primary and the other secondary, based on specific rules set by the insurers.

4.5: Appeals Process and Patient Rights

When you receive an insurance denial for a medication or treatment, remember that it is not necessarily the final word. You have options and the right to contest their decision. Let me break down the appeals process in simpler terms so you can confidently advocate for your healthcare needs.

1. **Initial Steps in the Appeal Process:**
When your insurance company denies your claim, the key is to understand why. The denial letter is your starting point; it will explain why the coverage was rejected and will outline the steps to appeal. This information is critical for your next steps.
2. **Building Your Case:**
Collaborate with your healthcare provider during this stage. Your doctor can provide important documentation, such as medical records, scientific papers, or personalized letters, to explain why a specific medication or treatment is necessary for your situation. These records serve as the foundation for your appeal, demonstrating the necessity of the therapy.
3. **Submitting Your Appeal:**
Provide supporting papers and follow your insurer's rules for appealing. This often involves organizing your gathered evidence and submitting it in a timely manner. Yes, it involves paperwork and may appear difficult, but this effort could be critical in obtaining the therapy you want.

4. **Seek support as needed.**
Taking up an appeal can be stressful, but you don't have to do it alone. Don't be afraid to ask for help from your doctor, a patient advocate, or a loved one. These allies can help guide you through the appeals process, ensuring that you present the strongest possible case.

Remember that the goal of this process is to ensure that you receive the most appropriate care and treatment for your health. With effort and the correct support, you can effectively advocate for your healthcare rights and potentially overturn the insurance company's initial decision.

4.6: Medication Refunds and Rights

Let's talk about something we hope you never have to deal with, but it's good to be aware of it if you do medication refunds. You may end up paying more for your medications than necessary, whether due to a pharmacy error or a delay in filing your insurance claim. But don't panic; you have options.

Getting a Refund from the Pharmacy:
If there's been a mistake in billing and you've overpaid, most pharmacies have policies to correct it and issue a refund. This usually needs to be done quickly, often within 14 days or less following the purchase. Based on your insurance plan rules, it's important to check your receipts and speak up sooner rather than later.

Dealing Directly with Your Insurance:
If you missed the pharmacy's refund window, you can still contact your insurance company directly to explain the situation and request a refund for any overpayments. This approach may take longer, but it is worthwhile if you believe you have been charged incorrectly.

Practical advice: Always save your pharmacy receipts and keep track of your insurance claims. Identifying and correcting differences early on is key to avoiding overpaying for your prescriptions. You have the right to pay only what you owe, and both your pharmacy and insurance company have processes in place to remedy overcharges.

Insurance doesn't have to be a cause of frustration. With knowledge and a proactive approach, you can efficiently navigate your health insurance to optimize your drug costs.

Up next, we're diving into mastering money-saving strategies on medications. Trust me, you won't want to miss the savings tips I've got in store for you.

FURTHER READING FOR CHAPTER 4:
INSURANCE NAVIGATION

Centers for Medicare & Medicaid Services (CMS)
For a foundational understanding of health insurance basics and insights into primary vs. secondary insurance, visit the Centers for Medicare & Medicaid Services.
Available at: www.cms.gov

Kaiser Family Foundation (KFF)
Explore detailed explanations of health insurance topics including prior authorization, formularies, and the appeals process at the Kaiser Family Foundation, a leader in health policy analysis.
Available at: www.kff.org.

HealthCare.gov
For comprehensive guidance on navigating insurance formularies and cost savings, along with understanding your rights under insurance plans, check out HealthCare.gov. Available at: www.healthcare.gov.

National Association of Insurance Commissioners (NAIC)
Gain insight into the appeals process and patient rights in health insurance from the National Association of Insurance Commissioners.
Available at: www.naic.org.

Consumer Reports
For practical advice on dealing with medication refunds and rights, consider the resources available at Consumer Reports.
Available at: www.consumerreports.org.

CHAPTER 5:
SAVING MONEY ON MEDICATIONS

Here are some tips that will help you stay healthy and save money at the same time. When it comes to medications, learning the ins and outs can save you a lot of money. We'll talk about the debate between generic and brand-name drugs and show you how to get the same quality for a lot less money. It's easy to find the best deals on medications if you go with me on a shopping spree. I'll be covering a huge number of deals, coupons, and help programs that can cut costs by a huge amount. As well as why it's important to ask for alternatives and how having this simple chat with your healthcare provider can save you a lot of money. Get ready to learn how to handle your medications in a way that saves you money and makes your trips to the pharmacy good for your health and your wallet.

5.1: Generic vs. Brand-Name Drugs

When you visit the pharmacy, you may be given two options for the same medication: the brand name or its generic. Let's clarify some common questions, help you understand the differences, and explain why generics can be a smart choice.

What Makes Them Similar:
Generic medications are comparable to brand-name drugs as they have the same active ingredients, safety profiles, potency, dosage forms, route of

administration, quality, and intended use. It's like comparing two recipes for the same meal made by different chefs; the ultimate result is essentially the same.

The Price Gap Explained:
Why are generics often much less expensive, you ask? Well, generic drug manufacturers don't bear the initial costs of developing and marketing a new drug, which brand-name companies do. Once the brand-name drug's patent expires, other companies can create a generic version of the drug. This competition often results in cheaper prices, with generics costing roughly 80-85% less on average.

> **Hack:** Always ask if there is a generic version of your medication. Choosing generics whenever possible will drastically lower your medication expenses while maintaining quality and effectiveness.

By choosing generics, you're making an informed decision about your health and managing your healthcare budget more effectively.

5.2: Finding the Best Pharmacy Deals

Let's look at how you can get the best pricing for your medications. The cost of medications varies between different pharmacies, and a bit of savvy shopping might lead to big savings.

Price Comparison Tools:
Price comparison tools, such as GoodRx and SingleCare, provide real-time price comparisons between pharmacies. By entering the medication name, you can see where it is being offered at the lowest cash price

> **Hack 1:** Paying Without Insurance – Smart Shopping
> When paying out of pocket for generic medications, consider exploring prices at big retailers like Wal-Mart or wholesalers like Costco. These outlets often offer lower prices for generics, making them a cost-effective choice. They also provide services for pet prescriptions, which might be cheaper than purchasing directly from your vet. Doing a little homework to compare prices could lead to significant savings.

(without insurance) in your area, potentially saving you a significant amount on each prescription.

Leveraging Pharmacy Programs:
Larger pharmacy chains such as CVS and Walgreens have programs that allow them to search through their database of discount programs to find the best offer for each medication without insurance, including finding manufacturer coupons.

Considering Independent Pharmacies:
While big chains are everywhere, it's important to consider your local independent pharmacy. Independents frequently offer reasonable rates and a degree of personalized care that you may not find elsewhere. They're also more likely to offer specialized services, such as custom medication packaging, to make managing your medications easier.

> **Hack 2:** Utilizing Insurance at Preferred Pharmacies
> If you're using insurance to pay for your medications, it pays to know which pharmacies your plan prefers. Preferred pharmacy status can mean lower co-pays and overall costs. Check with your insurance company or review your benefits paperwork to identify your preferred pharmacies. Taking advantage of preferred status can optimize your savings, especially when filling brand-name or specialty medications.

The Mail-Order Option:
Mail-order pharmacies can be beneficial for managing chronic conditions and ensuring consistent medication delivery. They not only provide lower costs for larger orders, but they also deliver directly to your door, saving you time and hassle.

Remember, a little research goes a long way when it comes to finding the best deal on your medications.

5.3: Discount, Coupons, and Assistance Programs

Understanding how to reduce the cost of your medications can mean significant savings for your wallet. Let's break down the tools at your disposal to make medications more affordable:

Discount Cards and Coupons:
Discount programs and coupons can provide significant savings on medications, especially for those without insurance or whose insurance doesn't cover a particular medication. These programs can dramatically cut the cost of medications—for example, turning a $100 medication into something more manageable, like $40. If you need help with your medication costs, ask your pharmacy for help. Most pharmacies have partnerships with discount card providers to help you find the discount program that offers you the biggest savings.

> **Nuance:** It's important to understand that the prices reflected for these discount cards are typically manufacturer or NDC-specific. This is a common occurrence, which is why sometimes, the price is different from what is stated on the website or app of discount programs like GoodRx versus the price you get at the pharmacy.

Manufacturer Coupons:
These coupons are direct from pharmaceutical companies and are particularly helpful, especially for newer or brand-name medications that might otherwise be too expensive. Some offer free fills of medications, while others can be used as secondary insurance to cover the otherwise high co-pay cost of a higher-tiered brand-

> **Hack:** Take advantage of the convenience offered by larger coupon programs like GoodRx. They have a separate customer service department or number you can easily contact. These customer support teams can offer additional support, such as helping you troubleshoot price discrepancies. Don't hesitate to use these additional resources to help you save more.

name medication. These coupons can be found by visiting the manufacturer's website.

Patient Assistance Programs (PAPs):
Many pharmaceutical companies have programs specifically designed to support those who are unable to afford their prescribed medication, offering it at a discounted cost or even for free. Eligibility is usually determined by income, insurance status, and the medication required. Applying may need paperwork and proof of financial need. Still, your pharmacy team can help you navigate this procedure, directing you to programs such as Pfizer's RxPathways and Merck's Patient Assistance Program.

Government Assistance:
Beyond the private sector, various government initiatives assist those struggling with medical expenses. We'll discuss these initiatives in more detail in the next chapter.

Remember, if you are concerned about the cost of your medications, communicate with your pharmacy team. They can help you navigate the maze of discounts, coupons, and assistance programs.

> **Hack:** For more resources on how to save on medications and reduce the cost of medical expenses in general, visit NeedyMeds.org. It's a non-profit website that serves as a one-stop resource, with information on patient assistance programs, drug discount coupons, and rebates, as well as resources for free or low-cost healthcare clinics and other savings programs.

5.4: Discussing Alternative Medications

If you're facing a high co-pay or your medication isn't covered, don't hesitate to ask your pharmacist for alternative options. There might be a similar medication that's just as effective but at a lower cost.

Pharmacists can be invaluable in identifying these alternatives. If you express concerns about medication costs, your pharmacist can suggest alternatives, such as moving from a Tier 3 medication to a Tier 1 or 2 option that's covered by your formulary. With your consent, they can then contact your doctor to suggest the change.

Wrapping it all up…

Managing your medication costs doesn't have to be a difficult task. With a bit of know-how and the willingness to ask questions, you can find significant savings. Working with your pharmacist and communicating with your healthcare provider can help you find ways to get effective and affordable care.

> **Hack:** While your pharmacist can start the conversation about switching medications, contacting your healthcare provider directly can speed up approval. Your doctor may respond faster if you contact them directly, speeding up the switch to a more affordable medication option.

FURTHER READING FOR CHAPTER 5:
SAVING MONEY ON MEDICATIONS

U.S. Food and Drug Administration (FDA)
For information on the differences between generic and brand-name drugs and how generics are approved, visit the FDA.
Available at: www.fda.gov.

GoodRx
To find the best pharmacy deals and compare medication prices, GoodRx offers up-to-date pricing and discount information.
Available at: www.goodrx.com.

NeedyMeds
Explore NeedyMeds for a wide range of information on discounts, coupons, and pharmaceutical assistance programs that can help reduce medication costs.
Available at: www.needymeds.org.

Consumer Reports
For insights into alternative medications and strategies to save on prescription drugs, Consumer Reports provides valuable advice.
Available at: www.consumerreports.org.

CHAPTER 6:
GOVERNMENT HEALTH PROGRAMS

Let's jump into the world of government programs together and learn how to use Medicare, Medicaid, CHIP, and VA Health Care! These programs can be life-changing, offering a range of benefits to meet your healthcare needs, but understanding them can sometimes feel like solving a complex puzzle. We're going to talk about Medicare Part D, explain what it covers, and how it can help your health journey. Learn everything you need to know about Medicaid and CHIP to make sure you and your family can get the healthcare services they need. For our veterans, we'll talk about the details of VA Health Care and how to get the most out of these perks. I'll also guide you through State Pharmaceutical Assistance Programs (SPAPs) and the 340B Program to show you how they can help you save a lot of money on your medications. It doesn't have to be hard to figure out how to use these government programs. If you have the right information, you can get a lot of health perks and help. Let's start this trip together, breaking down what seems complex and turning it into your stepping stone for better health and savings!

6.1: Medicare, Medicaid, CHIP, and VA Overview

Medicare Part D
Medicare is primarily a health insurance program for people over 65 and younger people with certain diseases or impairments, such as end-stage renal

disease (ESRD). For many, Part D of Medicare can be a tremendous relief because it is specifically designed to help with the cost of medication.

If you're eligible for Medicare, you're eligible for drug coverage (Part D). It's offered through private insurance companies, so you'll have the option to choose. It's important to choose your plan based on what medications you take and your financial considerations.

Medicare.gov is an excellent resource for thorough information on eligibility, benefits, and enrollment. You may also call 1-800-medicare for individualized assistance. Remember that understanding your healthcare coverage can have a big influence on your health and finances.

Hack: Use the Medicare Plan Finder tool on the official Medicare.gov website. This online tool can help you compare Part D plans, making it easier to find one that covers your medications at the lowest cost. Also, if you're on a tight budget, look into the Extra Help program, which helps with Medicare prescription medication costs.

Hack 1: Each state maintains a formulary or list of covered medications. Checking this list will help you determine which medications are covered. If your prescribed medication is not on the list, don't worry. Ask your doctor about prescribing a covered alternative or about requesting a Medicaid formulary exception. This means they'll ask Medicaid to cover your specific medication even if it's not on the formulary, especially if it's medically necessary.

Hack2: Another useful tip is to look into Medicaid's Managed Care plans if your state offers them. These plans may include additional benefits and medication coverage options. In addition, several states have support programs to help you navigate the Medicaid system, giving you specific counsel and helping you to maximize your coverage.

Medicaid

Medicaid serves low-income individuals and families, children, pregnant women, the elderly, and those with disabilities. The eligibility criteria vary by state since the federal and state governments jointly fund the program, but they generally consider income, family size, and disability status.

Medicaid's website for your state and healthcare.gov are excellent starting points for eligibility criteria, benefits, and enrollment processes.

Applying for Medicaid could significantly decrease healthcare costs, including prescription medications. Always keep up to date on your state's specific Medicaid options since they can change and even offer new benefits.

DUAL ELIGIBLES – MEDICARE PART D AND MEDICAID COMBINED

If you qualify for both Medicare and Medicaid, you have a unique advantage when it comes to covering your healthcare and prescription drug needs.

Medicare Part D is your go-to plan for prescription drugs if enrolled in Medicare. Now, Medicaid is a bit different. It's there to help people with lower incomes cover their health costs. It usually covers a wide range of health services, including prescriptions.

> **Hack 1:** One lesser-known benefit of the VA healthcare system is its mail-order pharmacy. It's really convenient, particularly for veterans who live far from VA medical facilities or have mobility issues. The VA mail-order pharmacy can deliver prescriptions straight to your home, saving you time and money. Furthermore, managing prescriptions through the VA's web portal or mobile app makes it easier to get refills and manage medication history. This program improves access to necessary medications and ensures continuous care, particularly for chronic conditions.

> **Hack 2:** Depending on your priority group, you may be eligible for reduced or no-cost copays. It's worth verifying your eligibility and enrolling in the proper priority group to reduce out-of-pocket costs. If you are experiencing financial difficulties, the VA provides assistance programs to help with prescription co-pays. Make sure to discuss your case with a VA social worker, who will walk you through the application process for these benefits.

> **Hack 3:** If your VA provider recommends OTC medications, ask them to write you a prescription. This will allow you to get them from the VA pharmacy or receive them through mail-order at no cost.

Here's where it gets good: If you're eligible for both Medicare and Medicaid (we call folks like you "dual eligibles"), you're in a pretty sweet spot. Medicare Part D pays first, then Medicaid steps in to cover any extra costs that Medicare doesn't, such as certain medications or co-pays. Plus, being dual eligible means you automatically get Extra Help under Medicare Part D. This means lower prescription costs, premiums, and co-pays.

So, if you're navigating both Medicare and Medicaid, know that they work together to keep you covered. It's like having a healthcare tag team in your corner, making sure you get the care and medications you need without the stress of high costs.

> **Hack 1:** CHIP also has a formulary. If the medication prescribed isn't covered, reach out to your pediatrician or family doctor. They can either switch to a covered alternative or help you apply for a formulary exception. This process could cover the original prescription by providing evidence of its medical necessity.

> **Hack 2:** Because CHIP programs differ by state, become acquainted with the advantages and enrollment dates relevant to your state. Some states treat CHIP as an extension of their Medicaid program, while others have separate or merged CHIP programs. Knowing the ins and outs of your state's CHIP program can help you maximize the benefits available to your child.

Children's Health Insurance Program (CHIP)

The Children's Health Insurance Program (CHIP) is an important program that helps children of families whose incomes are too high to be eligible for Medicaid but too low to pay for private insurance. CHIP covers a wide range of services, such as routine checkups, immunizations, doctor visits, prescription drugs, dental and vision care, to name a few, and even emergency services. It's a program that helps children receive the healthcare they require for a healthy start in life.

The official CHIP website in your state, which is generally accessible through the state health department's website, as well as InsureKidsNow.gov, is a good resource for learning about eligibility requirements, benefits, and application procedures. Remember that using CHIP coverage for your children's prescriptions ensures they have access to necessary medications and helps you manage your family's healthcare costs effectively.

VA Health Care
The VA healthcare system is a network that provides millions of veterans with a wide range of medical, surgical, and rehabilitation services. Enrolling in the VA healthcare system can provide veterans with access to medications, doctor visits, mental health services, hospitalization, and other benefits for a low or no cost, depending on various factors like service history, disability status, and income levels.

The VA's official website (va.gov) is a helpful resource for learning more about the VA healthcare system, eligibility, and benefits. Local VA hospitals and clinics are also available to help with enrollment and answer any concerns you may have about receiving the care and services you need.

6.2: State Pharmaceutical Assistance Programs

State Pharmaceutical Assistance Programs (SPAPs) aim to provide financial support to eligible individuals for prescription medications. They typically focus on seniors, those with disabilities, and low-income residents. These state-specific programs provide a variety of benefits, including covering co-pays, deductibles, and even medications not covered by Medicare Part D.

Eligibility criteria for SPAPs can vary greatly by state. In general, they consider age, residency, income level, and current Medicare Part D or Medicaid coverage. To find out if you qualify and how to enroll, visit your state's health department website or contact your local health services office.

Your state's health department is a wealth of information about SPAP eligibility and application processes. Additionally, Medicare.gov and Medicaid.gov offer information on how SPAPs work with federal programs.

IMPORTANT CONSIDERATIONS

Timing is Key:
Keep an eye on SPAP enrollment times to avoid missing out on potential benefits. These times may not always coincide with Medicare Part D enrollment periods.

Documentation:
To make the application process go more smoothly, prepare any relevant documentation ahead of time, such as income verification, Medicare or Medicaid information, and medical prescriptions.

> **Hack:** If you have Medicare Part D, SPAPs can help you cover costs that Part D does not cover. It's a good idea to find out how the two can work together to your advantage. SPAPs may provide additional support where Medicaid falls short, particularly in states where Medicaid prescription coverage is limited.

State pharmaceutical assistance programs (SPAPs) provide an important support system for managing prescription costs, especially for people currently on Medicare Part D or Medicaid. While the regulations and benefits of SPAPs differ by state, understanding these programs can result in significant savings and peace of mind.

6.3: The 340B Drug Pricing Program

Imagine stepping into a pharmacy and finding that your prescription costs are much lower than they would be elsewhere. That's the power of the 340B Drug Pricing Program, a little-known gem in the healthcare system.

> **Hack:** Anyone is eligible, regardless of income, as long as they are seen at a 340B participating facility, are seen by a 340B healthcare provider in that facility, and fill their prescription at a 340B contracted pharmacy, which is often attached to or near the 340B participating facility.

The 340B Drug Pricing Program is a federal program established under Section 340B of the Public Health

Service Act that helps people in underserved communities or those struggling with medication costs to access their prescriptions at a lower price. The program is administered by The Health Resources and Services Administration (HRSA), which is part of the U.S. Department of Health and Human Services (HHS). It provides benefits to individuals regardless of their insurance status. Additionally, depending on the program, other resources such as health screenings, free vaccinations, patient education, and counseling may also be available to those who need them.

Who Gets the Benefits?

It is primarily intended for people receiving outpatient care from certain hospitals and clinics, particularly those in rural areas that serve a large number of low-income, uninsured, and even undocumented patients. These healthcare providers can acquire medications at significantly cheaper prices and pass the savings on to you. It's especially useful for managing chronic conditions like diabetes or HIV/AIDS, where medication costs can quickly add up.

Finding the Right Place for Your Prescriptions:

The first step is to identify healthcare providers, hospitals, or clinics that participate in the 340B program. These entities can be found using the HRSA website, using their Find a Health Center link. Make an appointment and during your appointment, discuss your medication needs and any additional support services you may require.

> **Hack:** To get the best discounts, fill your prescriptions at a pharmacy that participates in your healthcare provider's 340B program. You can often get medications at extremely inexpensive prices, including no co-pays. Some 340B participating Health Care Centers might have free health screenings or educational resources, so don't forget to ask about what's available.

Your healthcare provider can guide you through the process and help you effectively access the benefits of the 340B program.

For those interested in learning more about the ins and outs of the program or digging deeper, The Health Resources and Services Administration

(HRSA), which supervises the 340B program, has a wealth of information on its website. In addition, 340B Health, an organization for providers in the program, offers resources that can help you navigate the system.

The 340B Program allows eligible healthcare organizations and covered entities to purchase medications at much lower costs. It's designed to stretch limited federal resources to provide more comprehensive services and reach more patients. While patients don't sign up directly for this program, asking your healthcare provider if they participate can result in lower costs on medications and other healthcare benefits.

Wrapping it all up...

By understanding and leveraging these government programs, you can significantly reduce your prescription drug expenses.

Up next, we're venturing into the world of over-the-counter medications. There's a lot more to it than just picking up a bottle off the shelf, and I'll guide you through how to make informed choices for you and your family. Stay tuned!

FURTHER READING FOR CHAPTER 6:
GOVERNMENT HEALTH PROGRAMS

Centers for Medicare & Medicaid Services (CMS)
For an overview of Medicare, Medicaid, CHIP, and VA programs, as well as detailed program eligibility and benefits, visit the CMS website.
Available at: www.cms.gov.

Medicare.gov
Specifically for Medicare-related information, including coverage details and updates, Medicare.gov is the official U.S. government site for Medicare.
Available at: www.medicare.gov.

Health Resources and Services Administration (HRSA)
For comprehensive details on the 340B Drug Pricing Program, which allows access to reduced price medication in healthcare facilities, check out the HRSA site.
Available at: www.hrsa.gov.

National Council on Aging (NCOA)
To learn more about State Pharmaceutical Assistance Programs and other support available for seniors, visit the National Council on Aging.
Available at: www.ncoa.org.

CHAPTER 7:
OVER-THE-COUNTER (OTC) MEDICATIONS

Come with me into the world of over-the-counter (OTC) medications, where picking the right one is both an art and a science. There's more to over-the-counter (OTC) medications than meets the eye. They can be a quick and effective way to treat common problems like seasonal allergies and the odd headache. We'll take the mystery out of the shelves of choices by focusing on what to think about when picking the best OTC products for your needs. I'll give you secret tips on how to deal with common health problems and let you know when an over-the-counter (OTC) treatment is enough and when you should see a doctor. We'll also go into detail about common illnesses and then match them with OTC treatments that can help. This way, you can feel confident and well-informed about your choices. If you know what to look for, it can be easy to choose which OTC product to pick up. This will allow you to take care of your health in an effective and smart way.

7.1: Understanding OTC Medications

Over-the-counter (OTC) medications are excellent allies for controlling common health conditions without a prescription. They include pain medications, antihistamines, topical treatments, and digestive assistance. However, with great power comes great responsibility; making wise decisions for both safety and effectiveness is essential.

PRO Tip: Always start by identifying your symptoms accurately. This will help you limit your selections and find the medication that best fits your needs.

7.2 Key Considerations for OTC Use

Read the Label:
It might seem obvious, but the label is packed with important information. Look for the active ingredients, intended use, dosage, directions, and any warnings that may apply to your specific situation.

Know the Active Ingredients:
Many OTC treatments, particularly cold and flu drugs, have multiple active ingredients. Be careful of what you're taking to prevent doubling up on the same ingredients from different products, which could result in an overdose.

Check for Interactions:
If you are currently taking prescription medications, vitamins, or other OTC products, check for unwanted interactions. When in doubt, ask your pharmacist.

Consider Your Health Conditions:
Some over-the-counter medications may not be appropriate for certain medical conditions such as high blood pressure or diabetes. Decongestants, for example, can raise blood pressure, which would mean an alternative should be considered.

Lifestyle and Dietary Factors:
Believe it or not, your food and lifestyle might affect the effectiveness of certain over-the-counter medications. Antacids, for example, don't work as well when paired with spicy and greasy foods.

7.3: OTC Remedies for Common Issues

If you've ever stood in front of a large selection of healthcare products, feeling overwhelmed by the options and confused by labels, you're not alone. My goal is to turn that confusion into clarity so you can feel secure and knowledgeable every time you go for an OTC remedy. Over the years, I've had countless conversations across the pharmacy counter, all of which reveal a common thread: the desire for rapid, safe, and effective relief from minor health conditions that disrupt our daily lives. Here's a simple list to help you feel better sooner.

PAIN, HEADACHES, MIGRAINES

Remedies: acetaminophen (Tylenol), ibuprofen (Advil, Motrin), naproxen (Aleve), and Excedrin Migraine
Common Directions: Ibuprofen (Advil), 200-400 mg every 4-6 hours as needed; acetaminophen (Tylenol), 500-1000 mg every 4-6 hours; Excedrine, two tablets with water at the onset of migraine symptoms.
Considerations: Acetaminophen is friendlier on the stomach, although high dosages should be avoided to protect the liver. While ibuprofen and naproxen are effective anti-inflammatory medications, they should be used with caution if you have kidney issues or are prone to stomach ulcers. However, because of their anti-inflammatory qualities, ibuprofen and naproxen may be more beneficial in treating migraines. Excedrin is used to treat more severe migraines. It's a combination of caffeine, acetaminophen, and aspirin, making the combination more effective than either ingredient alone.

ALLERGIES

Remedies: loratadine (Claritin), cetirizine (Zyrtec), fexofenadine (Allegra), diphenhydramine (Benadryl).
Common Directions: 1 tablet once daily.
Considerations: Non-drowsy options such as loratidine, cetirizine, or fexofenadine are ideal for daytime use. Diphenhydramine is better

for immediate needs. For the best results, start therapy a few weeks before allergy season. If you are having trouble sleeping at night, diphenhydramine, which can cause drowsiness, is a good choice. There are different options, and some work better than others, depending on the individual. For example, loratadine might work best for you, but another family member uses fexofenadine because loratadine doesn't work for them as well. It's important to try a few days' supply and determine which non-drowsy antihistamine works for you before committing to buying a large bottle.

NASAL CONGESTION

Remedies: pseudoephedrine (Sudafed), phenylephrine (Sudafed PE), Nasal sprays (Afrin).
Common Directions: pseudoephedrine (Sudafed), 30-60 mg every 4-6 hours; phenylephrine (PE products), 10 mg every 4 hours.
Considerations: These decongestants reduce swelling in the nasal passages. Pseudoephedrine is more effective than phenylephrine, although it can cause more jitteriness, increased heart rate, and elevated blood pressure. It is also restricted in some areas due to the potential for abuse. Afrin should not be used for more than three days in a row to prevent rebound congestion.

COUGH

Remedies: dextromethorphan (Robitussin, Delsym), guaifenesin (Mucinex).
Common Directions: Dextromethorphan (Robitussin), 10-20 mg every 4 hours or 30 mg every 6-8 hours; Guaifenesin (Mucinex), 600-1200 mg every 12 hours
Considerations: Dextromethorphan helps stop involuntary coughing, while guaifenesin helps loosen and release mucus/phlegm. Drinking water will help guaifenesin work more effectively. Avoid taking cough suppressants (dextromethorphan) at night if coughing helps clear mucus.

SORE THROAT

Remedies: phenol (Chloraseptic), benzocaine lozenges (Cepacol), Warm salt water gargle, Honey (>1yo).
Common Directions: Use as directed on the package.
Considerations: Phenol and benzocaine provide brief relief by numbing the throat. Lozenges are choking hazards for young children, so a warm salt water gargle is a safer option. With a mild sore throat, honey (in adults and children over one year) can be soothing and has antimicrobial properties.

FEVER

Remedies: acetaminophen (Tylenol), ibuprofen (Advil, Motrin).
Common Directions: Take ibuprofen (Advil) 200-400 mg every 4-6 hours as needed and acetaminophen (Tylenol) 500-1000 mg every 4-6 hours.
Considerations: Alternating between acetaminophen and ibuprofen can be beneficial, but consult with a doctor to confirm safety. Acetaminophen is a safer alternative for people who have kidney problems or are at risk for heart disease. Ibuprofen can provide longer-lasting relief, but it may be harsher on the stomach and kidneys.

MUSCLE ACHES AND PAINS

Remedies: ibuprofen (Advil, Motrin), naproxen (Aleve), Topical creams (Icy Hot, Bengay).
Common Directions: Topical creams containing menthol or capsaicin can be applied 3-4 times daily.
Considerations: Topical creams provide localized relief with no systemic side effects. They are perfect for those who do not wish to take tablets. Oral NSAIDs (ibuprofen and naproxen) provide more comprehensive relief for both pain and inflammation, but if you use them frequently, make sure to consider stomach protection, such as eating first or taking antacids.

ACID REFLUX AND HEARTBURN

Remedies: H2 blockers (Zantac, Pepcid), proton pump inhibitors (Prilosec, Nexium), and antacids (Tums, Maalox).
Common Directions: Antacids like Tums or Rolaids can be taken as needed, following the label for specific dosages. H2 blockers like famotidine (Pepcid) are 75-150 mg twice daily. PPIs like omeprazole are taken once a day.
Considerations: Antacids provide quick, short-term relief. H2 blockers and PPIs are for regular use. PPIs take a few days to kick in, while H2 blockers work within 30 minutes to 1 hour. Long-term use of PPIs can cause nutrient malabsorption and increased infection risk, so make sure your healthcare provider is checking for appropriateness of therapy regularly, commonly every 90 days.

CONSTIPATION

Remedies: Fiber supplements (Metamucil), stool softeners (Colace), laxatives (MiraLAX, Senna).
Common Directions: Take fiber supplements like Metamucil, one teaspoon in 8 ounces of water 1-3 times daily, or Docusate, 100 mg twice daily.
Considerations: Start with fiber and hydration. These improve bowel movements by bulking or softening the stool. Laxatives should only be used as a last resort due to the risk of dependence with long-term use.

DIARRHEA

Remedies: loperamide (Imodium), bismuth subsalicylate (Pepto-Bismol).
Common Directions: Loperamide (Imodium): Take 4 mg to start, then 2 mg after each loose stool (not to exceed 16 mg per day).
Considerations: Loperamide slows intestinal movement. It treats symptoms but doesn't fix the root cause. Avoid it if you have diarrhea from a bacterial infection because it can slow down your gut movement and make recovery take longer. Use it for temporary relief and stay hy-

drated. Reach out to your healthcare provider if you are experiencing long episodes of diarrhea.

INSOMNIA

Remedies: melatonin, diphenhydramine (Benadryl, ZzzQuil), doxylamine (Unisom).

Common Directions: Melatonin, 1-5 mg at bedtime; Diphenhydramine (Benadryl), 25-50 mg at bedtime.

Considerations: Melatonin is an effective sleep cycle regulator with no risk of dependency. Diphenhydramine and Doxylamine should be used mindfully, as they can cause tolerance and sleepiness during the day.

SKIN IRRITATIONS (ECZEMA, RASHES, INSECT BITES)

Remedies: hydrocortisone cream (Cortizone-10), calamine lotion, oatmeal baths.

Common Directions: Apply a thin layer of 1% hydrocortisone cream to affected areas up to 4 times daily. This reduces itching and swelling.

Considerations: To avoid flare-ups, use mild, fragrance-free moisturizers. Hydrocortisone should be used minimally, applied as a thin coating on delicate skin areas, and for no longer than two weeks at a time. Breaks must be taken for a few days to prevent tolerance, skin thinning, skin discoloration, or other side effects.

ATHLETE'S FOOT

Remedies: terbinafine (Lamisil), clotrimazole (Lotrimin).

Common Directions: Antifungal creams can be used as recommended by the manufacturer, typically 1-2 times per day. For athlete's foot, treat for 1-2 weeks after it resolves; for jock itch and ringworm, treat for 2-4 weeks; and if nail fungus persists after 4-6 weeks, consider taking oral treatment.

Considerations: These creams kill fungus directly. To avoid recurrence, keep your feet dry and clean and apply antifungal lotion as directed for up to 2 weeks after symptoms have gone away. Topical antifungals are beneficial in mild cases, but for more severe or resistant infections, medication taken by mouth may be required with a doctor's prescription.

YEAST INFECTIONS

Remedies: miconazole (Monistat), clotrimazole (Gyne-Lotrimin).
Common Directions: Depending on the dosage of the product, apply the cream or insert the suppository as instructed on the packaging, usually once a day at bedtime for three to seven days.
Considerations: Even if your symptoms improve, finish the entire course of therapy. Talk with your doctor if this is your first yeast infection. Since some products may leak, consider wearing a panty liner.

MOTION SICKNESS

Remedies: meclizine (Bonine), dimenhydrinate (Dramamine).
Common Directions: dimenhydrinate (Dramamine), 50-100 mg every 4-6 hours; meclizine (Bonine), 25-50 mg once daily.
Considerations: These lessen motion sickness symptoms. Although drowsiness is a typical side effect, taking medication 1-2 hours prior to travel can help prevent motion sickness symptoms. Meclizine is a preferable choice for people who need to stay awake. Dimenhydrinate is more effective but can cause more sleepiness.

MINOR BURNS AND SUNBURN

Remedies: Aloe Vera gel, moisturizing lotions (without alcohol), hydrocortisone cream for mild sunburns, NSAIDs (Ibuprofen)
Common Directions: Cool the burn by running under cool (not cold) water for 10-15 minutes; apply aloe or moisturizing lotion 3 to 4 times a day as needed until the skin is healed. For more discomfort and swelling, use hydrocortisone cream as directed on the package, typically up to 4 times a day.
Considerations: Burns can cause fluid to be drawn towards the skin and away from other parts of the body, so drink lots of fluids to aid in your body's recovery. Steer clear of more sun exposure. Keep the area

cool and moisturized. Avoid petroleum-based items as they may hold onto heat. Consult your healthcare professional for assistance if you have a severe sunburn that causes blisters, fever, or excruciating pain. Until the burn heals, keep it covered and keep it out of the sun. Use a non-adhesive, sterile bandage; stay away from fluffy cotton. Using NSAIDs can reduce inflammation and pain.

INSECT BITES AND STINGS

Remedies: hydrocortisone cream, calamine lotion, oral antihistamines (Benadryl, Claritin, Zyrtec, Allegra),
Common Directions: wash the bite with soap and water to prevent infection and apply a cold pack for 10-15 minutes to lessen swelling and numb the area. Apply hydrocortisone cream 1% or calamine lotion to affected areas up to 4 times daily to help with itching and inflammation. Take antihistamines as directed for itching and swelling.
Considerations: Oral antihistamines can help with itching; diphenhydramine works fast but may cause sleepiness. Non-drowsy antihistamines such as loratadine (Claritin), cetirizine(Zyrtec), or fexofenadine(Allegra) are better for those who need to stay alert. Keep an eye out for allergic reactions that may need emergency medical intervention.

DANDRUFF

Remedies: pyrithione zinc shampoos (Head & Shoulders), selenium sulfide shampoo (Selsun Blue), ketoconazole (Nizoral).
Common Directions: Ketoconazole shampoo (Nizoral) can be used every 3-4 days for up to 8 weeks; selenium sulfide shampoo (Selsun Blue) can be used twice a week for two weeks.
Considerations: These shampoos are designed to combat the dandruff-causing fungus. Use regularly to manage symptoms; switch up your shampoos if they start to lose their effectiveness. Ketoconazole is a strong treatment for dandruff caused by fungi, while selenium sulfide can also tackle the yeast component. Make your decision depending on the doctor's diagnosis of the type and extent of your dandruff.

HEMORRHOIDS

Remedies: witch hazel pads (Tucks), hydrocortisone creams, phenylephrine suppositories (Preparation H)
Common Directions: Over-the-counter creams or suppositories like Preparation H, use up to 4 times daily.
Considerations: These products help lessen itching, pain, and inflammation. Avoid sitting for long periods. While over-the-counter lotions and suppositories can alleviate symptoms, long-term therapy requires a change in lifestyle (more fiber in the diet and more water). Suppositories are better for internal hemorrhoids, whereas creams are better for external use. Wipes are helpful for both, primarily for hygienic purposes and temporary symptom relief.

WARTS

Remedies: salicylic acid patches (Compound W), freeze-off treatments.
Common Directions: Apply the solution or patch to the wart as directed, usually once daily.
Considerations: It may take several weeks to see results. Use petroleum jelly to shield the nearby skin to avoid irritation. The effectiveness of treatment depends on consistency; some treatments need to be repeated multiple times. Boosting the immune system by staying healthy can support the body's defenses against the wart-causing virus. To stop the virus from infecting other areas of the body or other individuals, do not pick or scratch the warts. Avoid applying treatments to your face or genitalia without first seeing your healthcare provider.

ACNE

Remedies: benzoyl peroxide (for killing bacteria and clearing pores) or salicylic acid (for exfoliating the skin and unclogging pores).
Common Directions: Start with the lowest concentration and apply once daily, gradually increasing to twice a day if tolerated. Apply a small amount to the entire affected area after washing. Moisturize as needed to combat dryness.

Considerations: These treat acne by killing bacteria or helping the skin shed dead cells. Although mild acne can benefit from benzoyl peroxide, it can be drying. Salicylic acid is kinder and aids in clearing clogged pores. When selecting from these alternatives, consider your skin type.

URINARY TRACT INFECTIONS (UTI)

Remedies: phenazopyridine (AZO), cranberry Products
Common Directions: Use as directed on the package, preferably after meals and at bedtime for up to two days. This should not substitute medical treatment from a healthcare provider.
Considerations: OTC remedies like phenazopyridine can only provide symptom relief and do not treat the UTI itself. It will also discolor your urine and stool into a brownish-red color. Cranberry products have been suggested to prevent UTIs, but they should not replace medical treatment. Keep a watchful eye on your symptoms. Ask for help right away if your symptoms increase, you have a fever, or you have back pain.

7.4: Consulting Healthcare Professionals

Even with the abundance of over-the-counter choices, there are situations in which consulting a professional is best:

Ongoing Symptoms:
You should consult a doctor if your symptoms don't improve or worsen, even after taking over-the-counter medication for a few days.

Chronic Conditions:
Your medication needs may be more complicated if you have chronic health problems like diabetes. A healthcare professional can offer tailored advice.

Medication Interactions:
Pharmacists can help to identify possible medication interactions between any new over-the-counter products you may be thinking about and your current medications.

Remember that over-the-counter medication aims to safely and efficiently treat common medical conditions. Make sure these easy fixes work for you by doing your research and choosing wisely.

FURTHER READING FOR CHAPTER 7:
OVER-THE-COUNTER (OTC) MEDICATIONS

Mayo Clinic – Drug Information
Offers comprehensive health information on the safe use of over-the-counter and prescription medications, including side effects and interactions.
Available at: www.mayoclinic.org/drugs-supplements.

WebMD – Medication Guides
Provides detailed guides on over-the-counter medications, including dosages, side effects, and when to consult a healthcare provider.
Available at: www.webmd.com/drugs/2/index)

U.S. Food and Drug Administration (FDA) – Over-The-Counter Medicines
The official FDA page on the safe use of OTC medicines, offering tips on how to read labels and understand drug interactions.
Available at: www.fda.gov/drugs/type-otc-medicines.

Centers for Disease Control and Prevention (CDC) – Healthy Living
Provides information on maintaining health and preventing diseases, including the responsible use of medications.
Available at: www.cdc.gov/healthyLiving/index.html.

National Institutes of Health (NIH) – MedlinePlus – Medicines
MedlinePlus offers reliable, up-to-date health information about medicines, covering a wide range of medications and their proper use.
Available at: medlineplus.gov/medicines.html.

Harvard Health Publishing – Harvard Medical School
Features articles on medications and supplements, providing insights into their benefits, risks, and management strategies.
Available at: www.health.harvard.edu/topics/drugs-and-medications.

The Merck Manuals – Consumer Version
Provides detailed, accessible medical information on drug use and how different medications can be safely managed at home.
Available at: www.merckmanuals.com/home.

CHAPTER 8:
NATURAL AND HERBAL REMEDIES

Let's have a trip through the green and leafy world of herbal and natural remedies. Nature's gifts can help you in many ways. In this chapter, we'll follow the natural road with an eye for detail and a dose of caution to find the safest and most effective ways to use Mother Nature's pharmacy. From the common cold to digestive discomfort, we'll match common ailments with their herbal remedies, giving you a toolbox of solutions that use the power of nature. And for people who like to do things themselves, we'll talk about do-it-yourself (DIY) remedies and show you how to make effective natural solutions right in your kitchen. We'll be covering the ancient wisdom and modern science behind herbal remedies, giving you the confidence and knowledge to embrace the natural path.

8.1 Using Herbal Remedies Safely

Let's set the scene with a few important things to remember before we delve into the world of herbal medicines for common disorders. This part of the guide will introduce you to natural alternative remedies that many find beneficial. Still, navigating through this section requires a bit of savvy:

Professional Guidance is Key:
Just because it's natural doesn't mean it's a one-size-fits-all solution. Since each person's health journey is different, it's important to speak with a healthcare provider before experimenting with new herbal therapies. They

can offer tailored guidance based on your overall health and consider any medications you currently use.

Understanding Regulation and Research:
Unlike conventional medications, natural and herbal products don't undergo the same strict regulatory processes. This means that the amount of medical proof supporting their safety and effectiveness may be limited. It is important to approach these remedies with knowledge, keeping in mind that the evidence may not be as strong as that of prescription medications.

Quality Matters:
The quality of herbal remedies available on the market can vary. Choosing remedies from reputable sources can help ensure the product you receive is safe and pure. Your greatest options are brands dedicated to quality and transparency.

Pay Attention to Your Body:
Pay attention to how every new treatment makes you feel. Reactions can vary widely from person to person, so it's important to listen to your body and adjust accordingly.

Determining Drug Interactions:
Determining drug interactions can be challenging when integrating herbal remedies into your daily routine. Due to not having enough studies and information, there may not be as much information available on how natural treatments interact with other pharmaceuticals. This emphasizes how important it is to speak with healthcare professionals who can help you through these uncertainties and ensure your safety.

Taking a chance on herbal remedies could seem overwhelming. Prioritize safety, take a cautious approach, and arm yourself with as much knowledge as you can.

8.2: Remedies for Common Health Issues

Whether you're suffering from insomnia or a persistent cough, there's probably a plant out there that can help. But keep in mind that, despite its awesomeness, nature's medication has certain drawbacks. Here is a summary of common illnesses and their herbal remedies in an easy-to-digest and even easier-to-remember format.

COMMON COLD AND FLU

Echinacea: Increases immunity. It can be taken as a tea or as a supplement at the onset of symptoms.
Elderberry: Its antiviral qualities help lessen the degree and length of the symptoms. It can be used as lozenges or syrup.
Why: Both herbs boost the immune system and may shorten the length of colds and the flu.
Considerations: Because echinacea can further stimulate the immune system, it might not be suitable for people with autoimmune conditions. Because raw berries can cause botulism, avoid giving elderberries to children under one year old. Also, make sure the items are from a reliable source to prevent toxicity. Results regarding how well they work are mixed and sometimes contradictory, which means more research is needed.

INSOMNIA AND SLEEP DISORDERS

Valerian Root: Acts as a natural sedative. Drink it as tea or take it as a supplement 30 minutes before bed.
Lavender: Known for its calming and sleep-inducing effects. Use essential oil in a diffuser at bedtime.
Why: They promote relaxation and help improve sleep quality.
Considerations: Interactions may arise when Valerian Root is taken with sedatives or other medications that affect the central nervous system. Alcohol should not be consumed while using Valerian Root be-

cause of its additive sedative effects. Although high amounts of lavender can be hazardous if consumed orally, topical or inhalation application is typically regarded as safe. Before using, women who are nursing or pregnant should speak with a healthcare professional.

DIGESTIVE ISSUES (BLOATING, INDIGESTION)

Peppermint: Relieve symptoms like bloating and gas. Drink it as tea or take enteric-coated capsules.
Ginger: Eases nausea and digestive discomfort. Use fresh in meals, as tea, or in capsules.
Why: Both have properties that help soothe the digestive tract.
Considerations: Babies and young children should not have peppermint oil applied directly to their faces since it could cause respiratory problems. Excessive intake of ginger may raise the risk of bleeding, particularly in people on blood thinners. If you take blood-clotting drugs or have gallstones, limit your intake.

ANXIETY AND STRESS

Chamomile: Has calming effects. Drink it as tea or take it as a supplement.
Ashwagandha: It is a remedy that helps the body adapt to stressors, reducing stress levels. When taken as a supplement, take it as directed on the packaging.
Why: These herbs help lower stress and anxiety levels through their natural calming properties, as well as help the body adapt to stressors.
Considerations: If you have a daisy allergy, avoid chamomile. Blood-thinning medications may interact with chamomile, increasing the risk of bleeding. Ashwagandha may interact with thyroid medicines and reduce blood pressure. It may also cause miscarriage, so pregnant women should avoid it.

ANXIETY AND STRESS (ADDITIONAL REMEDIES)

Passionflower: Has sedative and anti-anxiety effects. Drink it as tea or take it as a supplement.
Lemon Balm: Known for its calming effects. Use as a tea or in aromatherapy.
Why: They have natural anti-anxiety effects that help soothe the mind and help with symptoms of anxiety.
Considerations: Both passionflower and lemon balm can have sedative effects, which may interact with medications that make you drowsy, making it difficult to drive or operate machinery.

HEADACHES AND MIGRAINES

Feverfew: Prevents and reduces migraine frequency. Take as dried leaves, capsules, or tablets.
Butterbur: Reduces inflammation and migraine symptoms. This can be taken as a supplement under guidance, as it must be PA-free.
Why: They are thought to contain compounds that lessen inflammation and migraine frequency.
Considerations: If feverfew is stopped suddenly after prolonged use, it might result in withdrawal symptoms, digestive problems, and mouth ulcers. Additionally, it might interfere with some drugs, such as blood thinners like clopidogrel. Belching, headaches, itchy eyes, diarrhea, breathing problems, and exhaustion are some of the side effects of butterbur. In addition, you must talk to a healthcare professional before starting it, particularly if you have liver disease or are taking medication that the liver breaks down.

SORE THROAT

Slippery Elm: Forms a soothing film over the throat. Use as lozenges or tea.
Licorice Root: Has anti-inflammatory properties. Drink as tea or gargle.
Why: These herbs help soothe irritation and reduce inflammation in the throat.

Considerations: Herbs such as slippery elm and licorice root might cause allergic reactions in certain people. Pregnant women should use caution or stay away. For example, licorice root should not be used due to possible effects on hormone levels. Clinical evidence is limited and sparse for both.

HIGH BLOOD PRESSURE

Hawthorn: Supports the control of blood pressure and heart health. It can be consumed as a tea or as a supplement.
Garlic: It may have a reducing effect on blood pressure. Take it as a supplement or consume it raw.
Why: They may help lower blood pressure and improve cardiovascular health.
Considerations: Garlic and hawthorn can potentially interfere with the effectiveness of prescription medications for blood pressure or heart conditions. Clinical trials support the benefits of both hawthorn and garlic, although results can vary.

ARTHRITIS AND JOINT PAIN

Turmeric: includes an ingredient with anti-inflammatory properties. Use as a supplement or in cooking.
Boswellia: It is also referred to as frankincense and has anti-inflammatory effects. It can be taken as a supplement.
Why: These herbs can reduce pain and inflammation.
Considerations: If you take blood thinners, be aware of the possible blood-thinning effects of turmeric and boswellia. Long-term usage of turmeric tablets is not recommended because they can upset your stomach or lead to other issues.

SKIN CONDITIONS (ECZEMA, PSORIASIS)

Aloe Vera: Heals and moisturizes the skin. Directly apply to the region that is affected.

Calendula: Has healing and anti-inflammatory effects. Apply as an ointment or cream.
Why: These herbs help heal, reduce inflammation, and soothe skin irritation.
Considerations: Aloe vera and calendula are generally soothing, although some people may experience irritation or allergic reactions to them. Patch testing should always be done before applying to a larger area.

MENSTRUAL CRAMPS

Ginger: Helps lessen the degree and length of the discomfort. It can be used as a tea or taken as a pill.
Cinnamon: Its antispasmodic and anti-inflammatory properties lessen cramping pain. Use it as a spice, a supplement, or an ingredient in meals or drinks.
Why: These herbs have anti-inflammatory and pain-relieving properties.
Considerations: While too much of either might lead to stomach issues, both ginger and cinnamon can help reduce the pain of cramps. Because it thins blood, ginger should be used carefully by anyone taking blood thinners or those who have blood disorders. Since large amounts of cinnamon can be harmful, it is best to use it sparingly.

MEMORY IMPROVEMENT

Ginkgo Biloba: Enhances memory and mental performance. Take as a supplement according to package directions.
Rosemary: Enhances memory and concentration. Use the essential oil for inhalation or add fresh rosemary to meals.
Why: These herbs have a well-established ability to preserve the brain and enhance memory and thinking.
Considerations: Blood thinners and antiplatelet medications may interact with ginkgo biloba, increasing the risk of bleeding. People who have experienced seizures in the past should be careful when using ginkgo since it may cause seizures in those who are prone to them.

When using rosemary essential oil topically, dilute it first. High dosages should be avoided by women who are pregnant or nursing.

FATIGUE AND ENERGY BOOST

Ginseng: Known for its ability to boost energy. It can be taken as a tea or a supplement.

Maca Root: Improves energy and endurance. Add powdered maca root to smoothies or take it as a supplement.

Why: These herbs help increase energy levels and improve stamina, making them ideal for combating fatigue.

Considerations: Ginseng may interact with blood thinners, diabetic medications, and antidepressants. Additionally, it could make you sleepy, particularly if you take large amounts right before bed. Although typically harmless, the hormone-active properties of maca root may affect conditions that are sensitive to hormone changes. Start with a low dose.

HAIR LOSS

Saw Palmetto: Can help with hair loss caused by hormonal imbalances. It can be taken as a supplement.

Amla: The vitamins and minerals included in Amla (Indian Gooseberry) are rich and support healthy hair. You can eat amla fruit or massage your scalp with amla oil.

Why: Due to their high nutrient contents and hormonal balancing properties, both remedies can strengthen hair follicles and encourage hair growth.

Considerations: Saw palmetto can interact with prescription medications and hormone treatments. Before using, people with hormone-sensitive medical issues should speak with a healthcare professional. Although amla is generally harmless, those with diabetes or those taking diabetes medication should be aware that taking large amounts of the fruit can decrease blood sugar levels.

IMMUNE SYSTEM BOOST

Astragalus: It strengthens defenses against illness and guards against colds. Add dried root to soups or take as a supplement.

Reishi Mushroom: It lessens fatigue and strengthens the immune system. Take it as a supplement or use the powdered version in drinks.

Why: These herbs are well-known for boosting the body's defenses against infections and disease by enhancing the immune system.

Considerations: People with autoimmune conditions should avoid using astragalus, as it can worsen their symptoms. Don't use it without checking with your doctor if you have an infection. Immunosuppressants and blood thinners can interact with reishi mushrooms. In certain people, it could also cause nausea, dry mouth, or dizziness.

Nature's pharmacy is extensive and unique, with an abundance of herbal remedies for an array of conditions. Though using herbal remedies can be interesting and beneficial, it's important to proceed cautiously. You must do your homework due to the potential for interactions and allergies and tailor your choices based on personal preferences. Herbal remedies are not a one-size-fits-all solution. Because everybody is different, what works for one may not work for another. Inform your healthcare practitioner of all relevant information at all times, especially if you are currently taking prescription medications.

8.3: Home Remedies and DIY Solutions

In the realm of herbal and natural remedies, creating your treatments at home can be a rewarding and effective way to manage common ailments. Here are some safe and practical DIY remedies that go beyond just brewing teas. Here's how you can harness the power of nature with ingredients you might already have in your kitchen or garden:

Aloe Vera for Skin Irritations
Aloe vera is effective at treating burns, wounds, and other skin irritations. If you own an aloe plant, cut a leaf and apply the fresh gel straight to the affected region. This natural medicine can help reduce inflammation and promote recovery.

Honey for Cough and Sore Throat
Honey, especially Manuka honey, has antimicrobial qualities and is a good cough suppressant. A spoonful of honey added to herbal tea or diluted with warm water could help soothe a sore throat or cough. Its soothing effects can help with cough and sore throat.

Turmeric Paste for Inflammation
Turmeric has strong anti-inflammatory properties. To reduce swelling and discomfort, make a paste by combining powdered turmeric and water and applying it to inflamed areas or joints. For systemic benefits, add turmeric powder to your food or create a golden milk by mixing it with warm milk and a dash of black pepper to enhance absorption.

Garlic for Immune Support
Garlic, known for its medicinal properties, including boosting the immune system and fighting infections, can be crushed and let sit for a few minutes to activate its beneficial compounds. They can then be added to any meal. Eating raw garlic can be potent, so incorporating it into meals can make it more palatable while still reaping its health benefits.

Apple Cider Vinegar for Digestive Health
Apple cider vinegar (ACV) helps improve digestion and manage blood sugar levels. To improve digestive function, mix a spoonful of ACV with a glass of water and drink before each meal. ACV can also be applied topically to promote skin health and rinsed through the hair to clarify and add shine. Some evidence supports its use in improving digestion and managing blood sugar, but more research is needed.

Coconut Oil for Oral Health
Coconut oil is said to improve dental health and remove toxins from the body. Swish coconut oil in your mouth for up to 15 minutes before brushing your teeth to help reduce bacteria, freshen your breath, and boost gum health. Known for its antimicrobial properties; but claims about detoxifying the body are less scientifically supported.

Lavender Essential Oil for Relaxation
Lavender oil is known for its calming and relaxing properties. Add a few drops to a diffuser or combine with a carrier oil such as almond or jojoba oil before applying topically to the wrists or temples to help decrease tension and promote sleep.

Ginger Compress for Muscle Pain
Grate some fresh ginger and wrap it in a cloth. Boil water, soak the cloth in ginger, and apply the warm compress to sensitive regions to help ease pain and reduce inflammation. Ginger has anti-inflammatory properties, but evidence supporting ginger for muscle pain is limited.

Oatmeal Bath for Skin Soothing
An oatmeal soak helps soothe itchy or irritated skin. Grind plain oatmeal in a blender until finely ground, then add to a lukewarm bath. Soaking in this mixture can help treat eczema, psoriasis, and dry, itchy skin.

Peppermint Oil for Headache Relief
Applying peppermint oil topically can help relieve headaches. For cooling relief, mix a few drops of essential peppermint oil and gently massage it into your temples, forehead, and back of neck.

Chamomile Ice Cubes for Skin Inflammation
Brew a strong chamomile tea, let it cool, and pour it into ice cube trays. Once frozen, wrap a chamomile ice cube in a cloth and apply it to inflamed or sunburned skin for a soothing effect.

Cinnamon for Blood Sugar Control

Cinnamon is known for its potential to help control blood sugar levels. To reap its health advantages, sprinkle it on foods or incorporate it into beverages. You may also boil cinnamon sticks in water to make a tasty tea that helps control blood sugar.

Salt Water Gargle for Sore Throat

A simple saltwater gargle might help relieve a sore throat and minimize swelling. Gargle and spit a mix of half a teaspoon of salt in a cup of warm water for a few seconds. Repeat as many times per day as necessary.

Baking Soda for Acid Reflux

Baking soda can neutralize stomach acid, providing immediate relief from acid reflux. To relieve discomfort, mix half a teaspoon of baking soda and water and sip slowly.

These homemade cures provide natural solutions for a variety of health issues. While they can be useful, they should be used with caution and in conjunction with professional medical advice, especially for serious or persistent conditions. Always think about your own health needs and, if required, seek advice from a healthcare professional.

FURTHER READING
FOR NATURAL REMEDIES AND MEDICATIONS

National Institutes of Health (NIH) – National Center for Complementary and Integrative Health
Provides comprehensive information on various natural remedies, their effectiveness, safety profiles, and clinical study findings.
Available at: nccih.nih.gov.

WebMD
Provides valuable health information, tools for managing health, and support to those who seek information. You can delve into details about both OTC and prescription medications and natural supplements.
Available at: www.webmd.com.

American Botanical Council
Features herbal medicine information, including comprehensive data on herbs, their health benefits, and usage precautions.
Available at: www.herbalgram.org.

Healthline
Offers accessible articles on the benefits and risks of various dietary supplements and natural remedies, along with tips for healthy living.
Available at: www.healthline.com.

The American Migraine Foundation
Provides specific information about natural remedies used in the treatment of migraines and headaches.
Available at: americanmigrainefoundation.org.

Mayo Clinic – Drugs and Supplements
Offers user-friendly information on medications, including detailed descriptions of drug interactions and side effects.
Available at: www.mayoclinic.org/drugs-supplements.

National Center for Complementary and Integrative Health (NCCIH)

Offers evidence-based information on various natural remedies and their effects, including herbs and supplements for different health conditions. Available at:www.nccih.nih.gov.

CHAPTER 9:
DIETARY INTERACTIONS WITH MEDICATIONS

Let's combine the fields of diet and medications since what you eat can directly affect how well your medications work. In this chapter, I'll show you how the right foods can work with your medications to improve your health and well-being. Let's talk about the most common situations where food and medications come together, spotlighting interactions that can help or hinder your treatment. Enjoy some useful tips that will make managing your food and medications easier and smarter. You can make your daily routine a health-boosting powerhouse by planning your meals around your medication doses or choosing foods that make medications work better. By joining me, you'll learn how to make your plate and pillbox work together for your health.

9.1: Nutritional Impacts on Medications

Believe it or not, what you eat and drink can have a big effect on how well your medications work. It's important to find the right mix to stay healthy.

What Food Does to Help Your Body Absorb Medicine
When it comes to taking medication, eating can be both good and bad. For example, in order for the body to fully absorb the drug levothyroxine, which is used to treat thyroid problems, it works best when taken without food.

On the flip side, medications like ibuprofen and other NSAIDs should be taken with food to keep your stomach from getting upset.

How Vitamins and Minerals Interact with Medications

Vitamins and minerals, not just food, can also affect how your medication works. For example, Vitamin K, which is found in green leafy veggies, is known to affect the blood thinner warfarin. Consistency is key—sudden changes in your vitamin K, like eating more green and leafy vegetables than your usual daily intake, can make warfarin less effective. Meanwhile, calcium pills can make it harder for antibiotics like tetracycline to work, so you should wait a few hours before taking them together.

The Grapefruit Rule

The grapefruit rule is a prime example of food-drug interaction. Some enzymes that break down medications in your body can't work as well when you eat grapefruit, leading to potentially dangerous levels of medication in your bloodstream. Medications affected by grapefruit include some statins for cholesterol (like atorvastatin), blood pressure medications (like nifedipine), and certain anti-anxiety drugs (such as buspirone).

Mixing alcohol and medications is not a good idea.

Alcohol can make the drowsy effects of many medications stronger, like antidepressants, sedatives, and even some over-the-counter cold remedies, which can make it more difficult to move or concentrate. Long-term alcohol use can also affect the metabolism or breakdown of medications, altering how safe and effective they are.

9.2: Food and Medication Interactions

Let's talk more about food and drug interactions by going over some common interactions and how to deal with them.

Calcium-rich food/Dairy vs. Antibiotics:

Do you love your morning cereal? If you're taking antibiotics like tetracycline or ciprofloxacin, you should hold off on the milk. Dairy can interfere with how your body absorbs these antibiotics, making them less effective against infections.

Fiber's Double-Edged Sword:
Fiber is fantastic for your gut, but it can also grab onto medications like levothyroxine, a thyroid medication, and lower how much gets into your system.

Balancing Fiber with Metformin:
If you take metformin to control your diabetes, you may need to take a closer look at a fiber-rich diet to make sure your blood sugar levels stay in check. Eating a lot of fiber can change how your body uses metformin, which could make it less effective. This interaction might not be significant for all, but should be monitored.

Tyramine-rich foods and MAOIs:
Tyramine, found in aged cheeses, smoked meats, and certain fermented foods, can cause dangerous spikes in blood pressure for individuals taking MAO inhibitors such as selegiline, a class of antidepressants. Avoiding these foods is suggested to keep high blood pressure from getting worse.

Magnesium's Timing with Osteoporosis Meds:
Are you taking osteoporosis medications like alendronate? Magnesium supplements can interfere, so time them apart to keep your treatment effective.

Licorice and Blood Pressure Meds:
Are you a fan of licorice? It could lessen the effect of your hypertension medications by messing with your sodium and potassium levels.

Caffeine and Asthma Medications:
If you take bronchodilators (Proair, Ventolin) for asthma, drinking too much caffeine can make you feel jittery by imitating and amplifying the effects of the asthma medications. While caffeine may have some impact, it's generally mild.

Caffeine and Stimulants:
Taking methylphenidate or another stimulant drug with caffeine can make side effects like nervousness, insomnia, and a faster heart rate worse. When taking these medicines, it's best to limit how much coffee you drink.

Protein and Parkinson's Treatment:
High-protein meals can affect how Parkinson's medication, like Levodopa, works, which could make them less effective.

High-Fat Meals and Certain Seizure Medications:
For individuals taking certain medications for seizures or fungal infections, such as Griseofulvin, taking the medication with a high-fat meal can make it work much better and make sure they get the best results.

Your pharmacist can help tailor advice to your specific needs, making sure your diet complements your treatment rather than complicating it. Plus, keeping a medication diary can help track any changes in how you feel with different foods, making it easier to spot and adjust for any interactions.

> **Hack:** Use WebMD's drug and supplement interaction checker to check for drug interactions between foods, drugs, and supplements. It is available at: www.webmd.com. Or Drugs.com's drug interaction checker which also allows you to input medications and foods to see potential interactions and their clinical effects, available at: www.drugs.com. Note that this should not replace the advice and guidance of your healthcare provider.

9.3: Dietary Management Tips

When it comes to your food and medications, it can feel like you're sailing through unknown waters. But don't worry—I'm here to help you stay on course. I'm going to tell you some smart ways to make it easy to take your meds and follow your diet. Let's look at these life hacks that can help your treatment work better and improve your health in general.

Master the Timing Game:
When you take your medication, especially with food, can have a big effect on how well it works. If you need to take medications with food, timing them with meals can help them work better and keep your stomach from getting upset. On the other hand, if you need to take your medicine on an empty stomach, try to do so 30 minutes before or two hours after a meal. This makes sure that your stomach is empty enough for optimal absorption. For example, thyroid medicines like levothyroxine work best when taken first thing in the morning, before food, so that the body has time to absorb them fully.

Write down your dietary journey:
If you're not sure how your diet and medications will affect each other, keeping a food log can help. Write down what you eat, when you take your medications, and any changes or signs you notice. This detailed record can show trends and interactions, which will help you and your healthcare team make the best changes for you.

Learn about the dos and don'ts of diet:
It can make a huge difference in your treatment plan if you know which things to avoid and which to eat. Some things can make the medications less effective, while others can help them work better. People who take blood thinners like warfarin need to know about vitamin K-rich foods and how they affect how well their medicines work. With this information, you can be sure that your health journey will go smoothly.

Plan Your Supplement Schedule:
If you're adding supplements to your routine, it's important to make sure you take them at the right times so they don't mix with your medications. Talk to your pharmacist about the best time to take supplements, especially if you are also taking medicines that may combine with them. Simple steps, like waiting a few hours between taking calcium supplements and some medicines, can help with absorption problems.

Use technology to help you:
In this digital age, you can easily find many apps that can help you keep track of your food and medicine needs. Use diet apps to help you make meal plans that work with your medications and medication management apps to keep track of your doses and set reminders.

Talk to Your Doctor Before Adding Supplements:
Before adding any new supplements, talk to your doctor first. Sometimes, "natural" doesn't mean "safe," especially when combined with prescribed medications.

Keep the lines of communication open with your healthcare team:
By telling your doctors what's going on, you can ensure that your treatment plan is changed in a safe and helpful way.

If you know what to do and have the right tools, you can easily navigate the complicated world of nutrition and medications. This will ensure that your path to wellness is well-informed and fits your specific health needs.

FURTHER READING FOR CHAPTER 9:
DIETARY INTERACTIONS WITH MEDICATIONS

Academy of Nutrition and Dietetics
For professional dietary management tips that consider medication use, explore the resources available at the Academy of Nutrition and Dietetics. Available at: www.eatright.org.

Mayo Clinic
Explore in-depth articles on drug interactions, medication management, and the impact of diet on medication efficacy. Available at: www.mayoclinic.org.

U.S. Food and Drug Administration (FDA)
Offers comprehensive resources on drug interactions, including those involving food and dietary supplements. Available at: www.fda.gov.

National Institutes of Health (NIH) – MedlinePlus
Provides valuable information on drug information, including how various substances interact with medications. Available at: medlineplus.gov.

American Heart Association (AHA)
Learn about cardiovascular drugs and how various factors including food can affect their effectiveness. Available at: www.heart.org.

Harvard Health Publishing
Find detailed discussions on how lifestyle, including diet, impacts medication effectiveness and safety. Available at: www.health.harvard.edu.

The National Center for Complementary and Integrative Health (NCCIH)
Provides evidence-based information on herbal supplements and their interactions with medications. Available at: www.nccih.nih.gov.

Drugs.com – Drug Interaction Checker
This tool allows you to input medications and foods to see potential interactions and their clinical significance. Available at: www.drugs.com.

CHAPTER 10:
PEDIATRIC MEDICATION MANAGEMENT

Welcome to the gentle but important world of Pediatric Medication Management, where your little ones' health is the most important thing. In this chapter, I'll walk you through the most important steps for picking out and handling medications for your child in a way that combines medical expertise with a parent's tender care. I'll cover how to choose the right medications so that they are effective, safe for children, and easy to give. I'll share insights on organizing and managing your child's medication regimen, turning potential challenges into smooth routines. I'll also cover practical techniques for giving children medication that will make the whole process less stressful for everyone. Plus, I'll provide strategies on how to make sure your child takes their medications as prescribed so that their treatment is consistent and effective. Let's embark on this journey to master how to properly handle your child's medications, giving you the information and tools to support your child's health journey.

10.1: Treating Common Childhood Conditions

In this section, we will explore common children's illnesses and use a combination of science, nature, and parental love to determine how to treat them.

COMMON COLD

Oh, the common cold! It's something that all kids experience. There is no cure, but comfort is king.

> **Hydration and Rest:** Have them drink plenty of water and give them time to rest. Staying hydrated thins mucus, and rest helps the body heal.
> **Honey and Lemon:** For kids over one year, a spoonful of honey with lemon in warm water soothes sore throats and coughs.
> **Nasal Saline Drops:** These are safe for people of all ages and gently clean out the nose. They also make breathing easier.
> *Considerations:* Children younger than six should not take over-the-counter cold drugs. Always choose polite and helpful care.

INFLUENZA (FLU)

The flu hits harder than the cold and needs more than just TLC.

> **Antiviral Medications:** Oseltamivir (Tamiflu) can make the symptoms less severe if started early, usually within 48 hours of the first sign of a cold.
> **Fever Management:** Take acetaminophen or ibuprofen to lower your fever and ease pain. Dosing should be based on age and weight.
> **Fluids and Rest:** Encourage your child to drink a lot of fluids and rest to help the body fight the virus.
> *Considerations:* Getting a flu shot every year is the best way to protect against the flu. Watch for signs such as trouble breathing or high fevers, which indicate that you should see a doctor.

INSOMNIA

When counting sheep doesn't work, and your child is tossing and turning, it's time to consider gentle but effective options.

Sleep Hygiene: Set a regular time to go to bed and make sure the bedroom is cool, dark, and quiet. Cut down on screen time before bed to help you get a good night's sleep.

Relaxation Techniques: Guided imagery, breathing exercises, or gentle yoga can help calm active minds and prepare for sleep.

Melatonin: Under pediatric guidance, melatonin can be a short-term solution for sleep issues, especially in children with certain conditions like ADHD or autism.

Considerations: Focus on the lowest effective dose of melatonin and use it sparingly and only under the supervision of a healthcare provider. When you notice sleeping problems have been going on for a long time, it might be time to get a full review to find out what's causing it.

STOMACH ACHE

Tummy troubles can turn smiles upside down, but with the right approach, your child can feel better sooner.

Dietary Management: Make sure your child eats regular, well-balanced meals and doesn't eat too much. If they have a slight stomachache, bland foods like toast, rice, or bananas can help

Warm Compresses: Putting a warm towel on their stomach can ease pain and relax their muscles.

Peppermint Tea: With parental supervision, peppermint tea can help with stomach problems and pain.

Considerations: Peppermint tea should be used with caution in very young or sensitive children due to potential of worsening of reflux. Monitor your child's symptoms and water intake to prevent dehydration. If your child has severe or persistent stomach pain, especially if other signs like a fever are present, get medical help right away.

HEADACHES

For kids with headaches, whether they are mild throbs or severe pains, it's all about balance and care.

Pain Relief: Acetaminophen (Tylenol) or ibuprofen (Advil, Motrin) can work as long as the right dose is given based on the child's age and weight.

Hydration and Rest: Headaches are often a sign that you need to slow down. Make sure your child drinks enough water and gets enough rest.

Cool Compress: Applying a cool cloth to the forehead or the painful area can help right away.

Considerations: If your child complains of headaches often, you might want to investigate possible causes, such as vision strain, dehydration, or stress. Medication should be used carefully to avoid overuse, which can lead to rebound headaches.

CONJUNCTIVITIS (PINK EYE)

Those pink, itchy eyes need gentle care to clear up.

Clean Compresses: Applying cool or warm compresses gently can help ease discomfort.

Antibiotic Eye Drops: These are used to treat infections caused by bacteria.

Artificial Tears: Lubricating eye drops that you can buy over the counter can help with dryness and discomfort.

Considerations: Keep your eyes clean, wash your hands often, and don't touch or rub your eyes. Pink eye is often contagious, so keep your child at home to prevent it from spreading.

EAR INFECTIONS (OTITIS MEDIA)

Ear-tugging is a telltale sign of an ear infection. Not all ear infections require medication, but all do require care.

Pain Relief: Ibuprofen or acetaminophen can help with pain. Following the right dose based on your child's weight and age is shown on the package.

Warm Compresses: Putting a warm cloth over the hurt ear can help your child feel better.

Antibiotics: Antibiotics, such as amoxicillin, are sometimes prescribed by doctors to treat bacterial infections.

Considerations: Finish all prescribed antibiotics to stop the infection from coming back. Keep an eye out for hearing problems or ear gunk coming out. Many ear infections are viral infections, so they won't need antibiotics unless specifically diagnosed as bacterial by a healthcare provider.

STREP THROAT

Strains of bacteria cause strep throat, which is more than just a sore throat and needs special care.

Antibiotics: Penicillin or amoxicillin are good choices because they kill germs and prevent complications.
Warm Saltwater Gargle: This can help older kids with throat pain.
Hydration and Soft Foods: Warm broths and cool drinks help soothe sore throats.
Considerations: Complete the full antibiotic course, even if your child's symptoms improve. Keep your hands clean because streptococci spread easily.

ASTHMA

Prevention and control are important parts of asthma treatment. Personalized plans are key.

Inhaled Corticosteroids: Using them every day lowers inflammation and asthma problems.
Rescue Inhalers (Albuterol): This helps quickly when your child's asthma starts to flare up.
Allergen Management: Keep your child as far away from known allergens like pollen, dust, and pet hair as possible.
Considerations: Keep regular check-ups so that medications can be adjusted as needed. Tell everyone in the child's life about their action plan for asthma.

GASTROENTERITIS (STOMACH FLU)

This stomach trouble can be a mess, but it's easy to handle with the right care.

Oral Rehydration Solutions (ORS): These are needed to prevent dehydration. Like Pedialyte, ORS replaces lost fluids and electrolytes.
Bland Diet: Once the vomiting stops, slowly add bland foods like toast, bananas, and rice to your child's diet.
Probiotics: These can help restore a child's gut balance. Yogurt or over-the-counter probiotic supplements are good options.
Considerations: At first, avoid dairy and sugary foods because they can make the symptoms worse. Seek medical help if signs of dehydration show up or if symptoms last for a long time.

CHICKENPOX

There are lots of itchy spots, but don't worry—this is just a phase that will end.

Calamine Lotion: This stuff helps stop the itching. Put it on spots gently to soothe the skin.
Cool Baths: Baking soda or flour added to bath water can help soothe red and itchy skin.
Antihistamines: Over-the-counter options like Benadryl can reduce itching and help with sleep.
Considerations: Cut your nails short to avoid getting skin infections from itching. The best way to avoid getting chickenpox is to get vaccinated against it.

BRONCHIOLITIS

This infection of the lower nasal tract happens a lot in babies and needs to be closely watched.

Humidified Air: A cool-mist fan in the child's room can help them breathe better.

Hydration: To keep from becoming dehydrated, encourage drinking small amounts of fluids often.
Nasal Suction: A bulb syringe or nose aspirator can help get rid of mucus and make it easier to breathe.
Considerations: Keep an eye out for signs of breathing problems, like fast breathing or breathlessness, that need medical help right away.

ALLERGIES

Oh no! My kid has sneezes, sniffles, and itches! For people with allergies, the key is to control and avoid triggers.

Antihistamines: Allergic reactions can be controlled with drugs like loratadine (Claritin) or cetirizine (Zyrtec).
Nasal Sprays: Steroid nasal sprays, such as Flonase (fluticasone), can help with swelling and are safe for kids to use for longer periods.
Allergen Avoidance: Identify triggers like pollen, pet dander, or certain foods, and limit your child's exposure to them.
Considerations: Keep the space clean, use air filters, and think about allergy tests for cases that don't go away so that treatment is more effective.

HAND, FOOT, AND MOUTH DISEASE

This infectious illness can be annoying, but it's easy to deal with if you know what to do.

Pain Relief: Acetaminophen and other over-the-counter pain medicines can help ease pain; make sure to follow the correct dose for your child's weight and age.
Mouth Rinses: You can make your mouth rinse with salt and warm water.
Cool Foods: Ice pops, yogurt, and cold drinks can help mouth sores feel better.
Considerations: Make sure your child drinks plenty of water and avoids spicy or acidic foods, as these can worsen mouth sores. Addi-

tionally, to stop the virus from spreading, your child needs to be clean and practice good hygiene.

LICE

Getting rid of these annoying little bugs takes time and effort.

> **Permethrin Lotion 1% (Nix):** This over-the-counter treatment works well when applied to the hair and scalp by carefully following the directions on the box.
> **Nit Combing:** Use a fine-toothed nit comb every day to get rid of lice and their eggs.
> **Essential Oils:** Tea tree oil, when added to shampoo, may help keep lice away, but it shouldn't be used as a cure.
> ***Considerations:*** Wash your blankets, hats, and clothes in hot water to get rid of lice or eggs that are still on them. Avoid overusing chemical treatments to prevent scalp irritation.

IMPETIGO

This bacterial skin infection needs to be treated immediately to prevent it from spreading and to help the body heal.

> **Antibiotic Ointments:** Mupirocin (Bactroban), an antibiotic ointment, is often used and left on the wound for a few days.
> **Hygiene:** Keeping the area that is affected clean and covering it with gauze to stop the infection from spreading.
> **Natural Remedies:** Putting honey or aloe vera on the areas can make them feel better, though they don't replace antibiotics.
> ***Considerations:*** Impetigo is very contagious, so make sure your child stays away from other people until they are fully healed.

SINUSITIS

Sinus infections can be difficult to treat, but with the right care, kids can breathe more easily.

Nasal Irrigation: Rinses or sprays with saline can help clear out sinuses.
Steam Inhalation: Another way to help clear up stuffy noses is to breathe in steam from a warm bath or shower.
Antibiotics: If bacteria cause sinusitis, your doctor may give you an antibiotic.
Considerations: Keep an eye on your child's symptoms and see a doctor if they get worse or don't get better in a few days.

URINARY TRACT INFECTIONS (UTIS)

UTIs need to be treated quickly to prevent complications and ease the pain of the symptoms.

Antibiotics: Antibiotics are the most common way to treat a UTI. A doctor will tell you what kind to take and how long to take it for.
Hydration: Drinking more water helps get rid of bacteria in the urinary system.
Cranberry Juice: Cranberry juice is often suggested as a way to avoid UTIs, but it shouldn't be used instead for medical treatment.
Considerations: It is important to finish all of the medications and see a doctor again if the symptoms don't go away or come back.

CROUP

When someone has croup, they often wake up in the middle of the night with a barking cough. It can be scary, but it's generally not too hard to handle.

Cool Mist Humidifier: These keep the air moist, which helps the child's lungs feel better and breathe easier.
Steamy Bathroom: Sitting in a bathroom full of steam can help, too.
Steroids: When things get really bad, a doctor might give you a single dose of oral steroids to help with the swelling in your lungs.
Considerations: To help your child breathe, make sure they are calm and standing up straight. If they are having trouble breathing while they are at rest, help them right away.

ECZEMA (ATOPIC DERMATITIS)

Eczema is a skin condition that causes itching. It usually doesn't go away and requires a comprehensive treatment plan.

>**Moisturizing Creams:** Using emollients regularly helps keep the skin moist and safe.
>**Topical Steroids:** These are used to stop flare-ups and help with inflammation.
>**Avoid Triggers:** Write down things that make your child's eczema worse in a diary or notepad to find and stay away from them.
>***Considerations:*** To avoid dryness and irritation, choose skin care products without scents and stick to a regular skincare routine.

TONSILLITIS

If your tonsils get swollen, either from bugs or viruses, the right treatment can greatly improve the pain.

>**Pain Relief:** Ibuprofen or acetaminophen can help lower fever and pain.
>**Throat Lozenges:** For older children, these can provide short-term relief.
>**Antibiotics:** If bacteria cause tonsillitis, antibiotics are prescribed to clear the infection.
>***Considerations:*** If your child is given antibiotics, make sure they finish the full treatment and stay hydrated with soothing liquids.

OTITIS EXTERNA (SWIMMER'S EAR)

"Swimmer's ear" is an infection of the outer ear canal that needs to be carefully treated to help relieve pain.

>**Ear Drops:** Antibiotic ear drops are often given to treat the infection, and steroids are sometimes added to lower inflammation.
>**Pain Management:** Pain medications that you can buy over the counter can help manage discomfort.

Keep Ears Dry: Earplugs or a shower cap can keep water from making the situation worse.
Considerations: Don't put anything in the ear canal, and make sure to follow the treatment plan exactly as provided to get better.

RESPIRATORY SYNCYTIAL VIRUS (RSV)

RSV is common in babies and young kids, and it can cause major breathing problems, so it's important to keep an eye on them and give them supportive care.

Hydration: Making sure your child drinks enough water helps the lungs work properly.
Humidified Air: A humidifier can help people who have trouble breathing.
Medical Monitoring: In the worst cases, the person may need to be hospitalized for oxygen therapy and more intense care.
Considerations: Since RSV is very contagious, it's important to keep the infected child away from people who are easily infected.

> **Hack:** Bookmark sites like the AAP and CDC for a treasure trove of parenting gold. They offer reliable advice on everything from medication dosages to when it's time to seek medical attention.

Treating common childhood ailments requires both understanding and care. Some health problems need to be treated by a doctor, while easy home remedies can improve others. Always talk to a healthcare provider to get a correct evaluation and treatment plan. Don't forget that your love and care are strong remedies in and of themselves.

10.2: Allergies vs. Cold and Flu

Figuring out whether your child has allergies, a cold, or the flu can sometimes feel like solving a medical puzzle. Understanding the differences between conditions can help you choose the best treatment. Let's look at the symptoms and signs that will help you tell the difference between these common illnesses.

ALLERGIES IN CHILDREN

Allergies are reactions of the immune system to normally safe substances, such as pollen, dust, or pet hair.

> **Symptoms:** Itchy or watery eyes, a runny or stuffy nose, and a sore throat are indicators of allergies.
> Unlike colds or the flu, allergies don't cause fever.
> **Duration:** An allergy child's symptoms will last as long as they are exposed to the allergen, which can be seasonal (like pollen) or year-round (like dust mites).
> **Onset:** Allergy symptoms start right away after being exposed to the allergen and may stay the same over time.

COMMON COLD IN CHILDREN

Viruses cause colds and happen more often in the winter, but they can happen at any time, especially with children because they are often exposed to group settings like schools.

> **Symptoms:** A runny or stuffy nose, sore throat, cough, slight fever, and general tiredness are some of the symptoms of a cold. Colds usually come on slowly.
> **Duration:** Cold symptoms typically last about 7 to 10 days, with the first three days being the most contagious.
> **Onset:** Symptoms usually show up after being exposed to the virus and get worse around day 2 or 3.

FLU (INFLUENZA) IN CHILDREN

The flu, caused by the influenza virus, is a more serious breathing problem than the average cold and is more likely to lead to complications. The potential for serious complications are higher for children and elderly. Medical attention might be needed if the symptoms don't improve or if severe symptoms like breathing issues happen.

> **Symptoms:** People with the flu have a high fever, chills, body aches, fatigue, cough, and headache. Children and adults alike may vomit or have diarrhea.
> **Duration:** Flu symptoms can last from a few days to two weeks, but they usually become less severe after two to three days.
> **Onset:** Flu symptoms are worse than cold symptoms and show up faster, usually within a few hours.

KEY DIFFERENCES AND CONSIDERATIONS

Fever and Body Aches: As for fever and body aches, they happen a lot with the flu, not so much with colds, and not at all with allergies.

Itchy, Watery Eyes: This is usually a sign of allergies.

Seasonality and Exposure: The time of year and whether or not the person has been exposed to common allergens or sick people can provide clues.

Response to Treatment: Antihistamines and staying away from allergens help with allergies, but colds and flu need supporting care and time to get better.

> **PRO Tip:** If you're a parent with a sick child and getting to the pharmacy is a challenge, take advantage of same-day delivery services for essential over-the-counter remedies. This option is particularly convenient for those days that you need treatments like pain and fever relievers, allergy relief, cough syrups, or nasal kits. However, it's important to note that certain medications, such as decongestants like pseudoephedrine, cannot be delivered due to stricter regulations. Always check with your pharmacy or neighborhood store for availability and restrictions on their delivery services.

You can get a better idea of whether your child has allergies, a cold, or the flu by looking at the specific symptoms when they start, how long they last, and how they react to different treatments. Talk to your healthcare provider right away if you're not sure about the diagnosis or if your child is in a lot of pain, has been sick for a long time, or is having trouble breathing. Your child will get better faster and more effectively if the problem is identified early and correctly.

10.3: Pediatric Dosing and Administration

Giving medications to children can feel like a tricky dance where you have to be careful and accurate at the same time. Here are some tips that will help you make this task a smooth part of your routine:

Dosing for Children
Children aren't just little adults; their doses are different and are often based on their weight. To get this right, we need to do a little more math. Take amoxicillin as an example. Its success depends on finding the right dose, which is important for healing and reducing side effects. To stay on track, always check amounts with your child's doctor or pharmacist.

How to Master Liquid Medications
It is important to shake liquid medications, especially ones that start as powder. Shaking them to a consistent mix is key. Get rid of the spoon. A dosing syringe is both more fun and more accurate and will help you get the right amount.

Tablet Tactics
If it's time to try taking pills, start with candy runs to get ready. Pill time can be a cool trick to show off with the "lean-forward" method for capsules or the "pop-bottle" method for tablets. If your child isn't ready to swallow them whole yet, see if you can break them up or crush them. But be careful because some pills, especially slow-release ones, are not meant to be altered.

Adding some applesauce to the bits can make the medicine taste so much better and go down easier.

Flavor Fun
The taste of medicine can be a deal-breaker, but flavoring services at pharmacies can make all the difference. Choosing a flavor that tickles your child's taste buds can make it easy for them to take their medicine.

Creative Taste-Masking
If adding flavor isn't enough, hide the taste with tricks. Adding a little chocolate syrup or peanut butter can cover up those gross tastes and make something taste good. Just make sure your pharmacist says it's okay before you mix.

Chilly Tactics
Putting liquid medications in the fridge can make them taste less strong. However, not all medications can be kept in the fridge. Pre-chilling your child's taste buds with something cold can also make the medication taste milder.

Gentle Desensitization
If your child is sensitive to taste, start slowly. Mix their medicine with their favorite drink, and then slowly cut back on the drink until they can take the medication without any problems.

With these ideas, you're not just giving medication; you're also giving care with a touch of love and creativity. You can help your child have a smooth and stress-free time with their meds by being patient and creative.

10.4: Medication Adherence in Children

Getting kids to look forward to taking their medicine is all part of being a parent. So, let's look at some cool ways to make the process easier and make sure your child sticks to their health plan without any mess.

Easy integration of routines
Adding medications to your daily routine can really help. If your child needs to take doses throughout the day, why not time them with important times like sleep or meals? For example, if they have to take amoxicillin three times a day, putting it at breakfast, lunch, and dinner can help them remember to take it, making it easy to stick to.

Good reinforcement works like magic.
Never forget how powerful a little support can be. A creative rewards system, like a star chart that builds up to a prize, can turn taking medications from something you dread to something fun.

How Curiosity Can Spark Change
Kids naturally want to know things. Use this interest to your advantage by describing the medication's benefits in terms they can understand. If a child with asthma knows that their inhaler is the secret tool that lets them play freely, it can really motivate them.

Getting used to technology
Apps and pill organizers aren't just for adults. These tools can really help you keep track of your child's medication routine and make sure that no treatment or dose is missed.

Games and Fun
Younger kids might like making their pill routine more fun. Make medicine time playful by using countdowns, personalized and painted medication containers, or a calendar full of bright stickers. This will make it a time they look forward to.

Using these tips can help you make taking medications a good part of your child's daily life. Open communication is key to managing your child's medications well, both with the healthcare provider and with your child and family members.

FURTHER READING FOR CHAPTER 10:
PEDIATRIC MEDICATION MANAGEMENT

American Academy of Pediatrics (AAP)
For guidelines on treating common childhood conditions and best practices in pediatric medication management, visit the American Academy of Pediatrics.
Available at: www.aap.org.

U.S. Food and Drug Administration (FDA)
For important information on pediatric dosing and administration of medications, including safety tips and guidelines, check out the FDA's resources.
Available at: www.fda.gov.

HealthyChildren.org
Explore practical advice on medication adherence in children, supported by pediatricians from the American Academy of Pediatrics, on HealthyChildren.org.
Available at: www.healthychildren.org.

Centers for Disease Control and Prevention (CDC)
A reliable source for information on infectious diseases, vaccinations, and public health guidelines.
Available at: www.cdc.gov.

Mayo Clinic
Provides detailed patient education material on a wide range of health conditions affecting children and adults.
Available at: www.mayoclinic.org.

KidsHealth
A resource for parents, kids, and teens; provides simple and practical advice on various pediatric health conditions.
Available at: www.kidshealth.org.

MedlinePlus – U.S. National Library of Medicine
Offers information on over-the-counter and prescription medications, health conditions, and management of diseases.
Available at: medlineplus.gov.

World Health Organization (WHO)
Features global health standards and information on the spread, prevention, and treatment of diseases.
Available at: www.who.int.

CHAPTER 11:
ELDERLY MEDICATION MANAGEMENT

Let's take a trip into the complicated world of managing medications for the elderly, where each prescription and pill is important in keeping them healthy and thriving. As we get older, our bodies and health care needs change, so the way we take medications needs to change, too. In this chapter, we'll talk about how to make better medication choices for the elderly so that they support a vibrant life rather than complicate it. We'll dive into the Beers List and find out what medications are best avoided or must be used with caution in older adults. I'll also cover the tricky area of using opioid painkillers and benzodiazepines together, with the goal of managing pain and anxiety effectively without putting too much at risk. Beyond prescriptions, I'll cover the benefits of integrating herbal remedies and over-the-counter solutions, offering a holistic view of elder care. As we work to make medication management easier for the elderly, we can make sure they are safer, healthier, and better informed about their health.

11.1: Managing Medications for the Elderly

Let's explore the world of managing medications for the elderly, where health, safety, and well-being are very important. I'm here to help you choose the right medications for our seniors and show them the extra care they deserve.

Navigating Age-Related Changes:
As we age, our bodies handle medications differently, making us more sensitive to their benefits and side effects. It's important to start with smaller doses and make careful adjustments, always monitoring for any changes.

Emphasizing Regular Medication Reviews:
It's important to talk to your doctor about all of your medications, even over-the-counter ones and supplements. This regular check-up can help find medications that should be cut back or stopped, like NSAIDs, which can cause stomach bleeding in older adults.

Opting for Senior-Friendly Medications:
Ease of use is very important. It can be very helpful for people who have trouble swallowing pills or are following complicated plans to have liquid forms, or only need to take them once a day.

Heeding the Beers List:
This important list shows which drugs might not be the best choice for people over 65, letting them know about possible higher risks like falling or getting confused. Talk with your healthcare providers about taking a medication list on the Beer's List. You might find better options that cause fewer side effects or are more effective.

Embracing Comprehensive Care:
Managing medications for the elderly is a team sport. Getting doctors, pharmacists, guardians, and family involved makes sure that everyone is on the same page about the medication plan and any special needs.

Leveraging Medication Management Tools:
From pill organizers to reminder apps, these are the best ways to keep track of your medicines, make sure you take them as prescribed, and avoid forgetting to take a dose.

Taking Care of Cost Issues:
The cost of medications shouldn't get in the way of care. Looking into generic drugs, assistance programs, or Medicare Part D can help with costs without lowering the standard of care.

By following these guidelines, we can improve the health and independence of our elderly and make sure that their medication journey is as safe and easy as possible.

11.2: Treatments for Elderly Ailments

Let's start our trip through the landscape of aging. By learning about and dealing with these 20 common illnesses, you can turn your golden years into a time of renewed health and vitality. Let's look at how combining modern medicine with natural knowledge can help seniors live happy and healthy lives.

ARTHRITIS

People over 65 often develop arthritis, which causes pain and stiffness in the joints. The best treatment is often a combination of medications and lifestyle changes.

> **Prescription Treatment:** Nonsteroidal anti-inflammatory drugs (NSAIDs), such as ibuprofen (Motrin) and naproxen (Aleve), can help relieve both pain and swelling. Medications like celecoxib or even corticosteroids may need to be prescribed for more serious cases.
> **Natural Approaches:** Glucosamine and chondroitin supplements, as well as omega-3 fatty acids found in supplements such as fish oil, are often used to help keep joints healthy. Ginger and turmeric are both known to help reduce inflammation.
> **_Considerations:_** Physical therapy, regular exercise, and watching your weight are all very important for controlling arthritis symptoms. When

taking NSAIDs for a long period, it's important to watch out for side effects such as gastrointestinal issues like stomach aches and to have regular kidney checks.

CARDIOVASCULAR DISEASES

Managing cardiovascular diseases effectively can improve the quality of life in older adults. This includes keeping high blood pressure, heart disease, and stroke under control.

> **Prescription Treatments:** Statins are often used to lower cholesterol, ACE inhibitors or beta-blockers are often used to lower blood pressure, and anticoagulants are often used to prevent strokes.
> **Natural Approaches:** Coenzyme Q10 and garlic supplements have been linked to heart health benefits. Eating fruits, veggies, and whole grains and maintaining a diet low in sodium are recommended and beneficial.
> ***Considerations:*** It is very important to monitor your blood pressure and cholesterol levels regularly and live a heart-healthy lifestyle. Be careful of possible interactions when you take herbal products with prescription drugs and the risk of bleeding with aspirin.

DIABETES

Controlling blood sugar levels is an important part of managing diabetes and preventing disease complications.

> **Prescription Treatments:** Metformin is usually the first drug used to treat type 2 diabetes, with insulin therapy being common in more advanced stages or for type 1 diabetes.
> **Natural Approaches:** What you eat is a big part of controlling diabetes. Natural supplements like cinnamon and alpha-lipoic acid have shown the potential in lowering blood sugar.
> ***Considerations:*** It's important to keep an eye on your blood sugar levels, eat a healthy diet, and stay active. Knowing when and how much

to take your medications in relation to meals can help you control your blood sugar better.

RESPIRATORY DISEASES

To keep a good quality of life and healthy lung function, older adults with chronic lung diseases like COPD and asthma need to be carefully managed.

> **Prescription Treatments:** Bronchodilators and inhaled corticosteroids are two of the most common medications used to treat COPD. They help open up lungs and lower inflammation. For acute flare-ups, **short-acting inhalers or systemic corticosteroids may be used.**
> **Natural Approaches:** While fewer natural remedies are available for respiratory diseases, practices like controlled breathing exercises and pulmonary rehabilitation are two examples that can help improve symptoms.
> *Considerations:* To manage these conditions, it's important to avoid things that irritate the lungs, stay on top of flu and pneumonia vaccines, and have regular lung function tests.

ALZHEIMER'S DISEASE AND DEMENTIA

Memory loss and the inability to do daily tasks are both affected by cognitive decline. There is no cure, but treatments can help manage symptoms.

> **Prescription Treatments:** Acetylcholinesterase inhibitors, such as donepezil, and NMDA receptor antagonists, such as memantine, are medications that are used to improve cognitive function or slow its decline.
> **Natural Approaches:** Ginkgo biloba is usually considered a way to improve brain function, but the results have been mixed. Antioxidants and omega-3 fatty acids are also considered helpful to brain health.
> *Considerations:* Keeping your mind active with puzzles, interactions with others, and regular exercise may help manage the worsening of symptoms. Making changes to the living space to make it safer and doing regular checks are important for caring for people with dementia.

RESPIRATORY DISEASES

Long-term breathing problems like COPD (Chronic Obstructive Pulmonary Disease) and asthma can make life very hard for older people. This is how we deal with these problems:

> **Prescription Treatments:** Bronchodilators such as albuterol and inhaled corticosteroids like fluticasone are the most common medications used to treat COPD. They are usually given through inhalers or nebulizers. Long-acting beta-agonists (LABAs) and leukotriene modifiers may also be used to manage asthma.
> **Natural Approaches:** Breathing routines, especially pursed-lip breathing, can help your lungs work better. Herbal supplements, such as ivy leaf extract, might help with mild respiratory symptoms.
> *Considerations:* Staying active with specialized exercises like swimming or walking can improve lung function. To avoid getting respiratory problems, it's also important to stay away from smoke and other pollutants and make sure that vaccinations are up to date.

OSTEOPOROSIS

This condition makes bones brittle, making them more likely to break. To strengthen the bones, we do the following:

> **Prescription Treatments:** Bisphosphonates, such as alendronate and risedronate, are often given to strengthen bones. Taking calcium and vitamin D tablets is important for bone health, but you also need to exercise regularly.
> **Natural Approaches:** To strengthen your bones, eat foods high in calcium and vitamin D, like leafy greens and dairy products, and perform weight-bearing movements.
> *Considerations:* It's important to test bone density on a regular basis to see how osteoporosis is progressing. Creating a safe environment to live in that helps avoid falls is also very important.

HEARING LOSS

To deal with hearing loss, you need to do more than turn up the volume; it needs strategic management:

Prescription Treatments: No medicine can fix hearing loss, but hearing aids and cochlear implants can significantly improve hearing.
Natural Approaches: Protecting the ears from loud noises can prevent further damage. There is ongoing research into vitamins and minerals that could support ear health.
Considerations: Getting your hearing checked regularly can help you keep track of changes, and helpful listening devices can make your life better. It's important to have Clear communication with friends, family, and healthcare providers.

VISION IMPAIRMENT

People often lose their vision, but there are ways to keep seeing:

Prescription Treatments: For age-related macular degeneration, treatments like anti-VEGF injections can slow down vision loss. People with glaucoma can use eye drops to lower the pressure inside their eyes.
Natural Approaches: Supplements with lutein and zeaxanthin, along with omega-3 fatty acids, are thought to help eye health.
Considerations: Getting regular eye exams is important for finding and treating eye problems early on. Having enough light and using magnifying tools for enlarging can help with daily tasks.

INCONTINENCE

While often overlooked, managing incontinence can greatly improve life quality:

Prescription Treatments: Medications like anticholinergics can help control an overactive bladder, while topical estrogen can help post-menopausal women with urinary incontinence.

Natural Approaches: Pelvic floor exercises (Kegels) can strengthen the muscles and help with leakage incidents. Bladder training techniques can also improve control.

Considerations: Making changes to your lifestyle, like drinking less alcohol and caffeine, can help with symptoms. Using absorbent products and scheduling regular bathroom breaks can also help manage the condition.

CHRONIC PAIN

Chronic pain, which often comes along with diseases like arthritis, needs to be managed in more than one way.

Prescription Treatments: NSAIDs or acetaminophen can ease pain, but opioids may be needed in more serious cases and should be carefully monitored because they can lead to addiction. Pain patches and topical painkillers can also help with localized relief.

Natural Approaches: Acupuncture and turmeric, which reduce inflammation, can be effective in pain management.

Considerations: Regular physical activity and physical therapy can strengthen muscles and reduce pain. It's important to find a balance between rest and activity and not to depend too much on medications.

INSOMNIA

Insomnia, the elusive sleep thief, can be tackled through various strategies.

Prescription Treatments: Sleep aids like zolpidem or eszopiclone are helpful for short-term use. For long-term effects, behavioral therapies should be added to these medications.

Natural Approaches: Chamomile tea, valerian root, and melatonin supplements are all well-known ways to help with sleep. Setting up a regular sleep schedule and a relaxing bedtime routine are also effective ways to deal with insomnia that don't involve medications.

Consideration: Avoid coffee and screen time before bed, and make sure your room is cool, dark, and quiet.

OBESITY

Addressing obesity requires a comprehensive approach in order to support long-term weight management.

> **Prescription Treatments:** Medications like orlistat can help in weight loss when combined with lifestyle changes. Newer drugs like semaglutide have been shown to be effective in obesity management, especially when combined with lifestyle changes.
> **Natural Approaches:** Eating a balanced diet full of fruits, veggies, and lean proteins is important, as is staying active every day. Behavioral changes, like eating more mindfully, can also have a big effect.
> ***Considerations:*** To improve your chances of success, set attainable goals and get help from a nutritionist or weight management program.

GASTROINTESTINAL ISSUES

Whether it's acid reflux or constipation, stomach problems need specific treatments.

> **Prescription Treatments:** PPIs, such as omeprazole or H2 blockers like famotidine (Pepcid), can help with acid reflux. Laxatives or fiber supplements can help with constipation, while antacids can immediately relieve heartburn.
> **Natural Remedies:** Ginger and peppermint are natural remedies that can help settle an upset stomach. Making changes to your diet, like eating more fiber if you have constipation or staying away from spicy foods if you have acid reflux, is also helpful.
> ***Considerations:*** Keeping a food log to find out what foods make your symptoms worse and eating smaller meals more often can help you manage your symptoms.

PARKINSON'S DISEASE

Parkinson's disease is a movement problem that needs comprehensive care strategies.

Prescription Treatments: The usual treatment is levodopa combined with carbidopa, which improves symptoms by replenishing dopamine. Based on individual needs, other drugs like dopamine agonists such as ropinirole or MAO-B inhibitors like selegiline may be used.

Natural Approaches: Exercise, especially yoga or tai chi, can help improve balance and mobility. Natural supplements are still being studied, but there is some proof that omega-3 fatty acids and Coenzyme Q10 can help.

Considerations: To effectively manage Parkinson's, it is important to get regular neurological exams, occupational and physical therapy, and participation in support groups.

INFECTIONS

Because their immune systems aren't as strong, older adults are more likely to get infections like urinary tract infections (UTIs), pneumonia, and the flu.

Prescription Treatments: Antibiotics are usually given for urinary tract infections (UTIs) and bacterial pneumonia. For flu, antiviral medications such as oseltamivir (Tamiflu) may be recommended.

Natural Approaches: Drinking Cranberry juice and taking probiotics can both help keep the urinary tract healthy and prevent UTIs. Elderberry and echinacea may help the body fight off colds and flu.

Considerations: Getting a flu or pneumonia shot is the best way to avoid getting these infections. Staying hydrated and practicing good cleanliness are essential to lowering your risk of UTIs.

SKIN CONDITIONS

Skin problems like eczema, psoriasis, and skin cancer need to be carefully managed.

Prescription Treatments: Topical steroids such as hydrocortisone or triamcinolone can help with itching and inflammation in older adults with eczema and psoriasis. When psoriasis is very bad, advanced treatments like biologics such as infliximab are used. Skin cancers may need to be removed surgically, with radiation, or with treatment.

Natural Approaches: Aloe vera, oatmeal baths, and moisturizing creams can all help soothe irritated skin. Keeping out of the sun and using sun protection is key to preventing skin cancer.

Considerations: Regularly checking the skin is important to detect changes early. Identifying and managing triggers like stress for psoriasis or allergens for eczema can prevent flare-ups

THYROID DISORDERS

Thyroid problems, like hypothyroidism or hyperthyroidism, can affect metabolism and energy levels.

Prescription Treatments: For hypothyroidism, levothyroxine is used to replace thyroid hormones that aren't working properly. For hyperthyroidism, methimazole and other drugs are used to control the condition.

Natural Approach: Iodine and selenium are important for thyroid health, but taking supplements should be done carefully and only with the direction of your doctor.

Considerations: It's important to check thyroid function tests regularly to adjust medication where needed properly. Diet and lifestyle adjustments are also helpful in managing symptoms.

KIDNEY ISSUES

Chronic kidney disease (CKD) can have a big effect on the health of older adults.

Prescription Treatments: Healthy blood pressure and blood sugar levels are important for older adults with CKD. ACE inhibitors and other medications are often needed to keep blood pressure under control. It has also been found to have kidney-protective properties.

Natural Approaches: Staying hydrated helps keep the kidneys working well.

Considerations: To manage CKD, it's important to get regular blood tests to check kidney function, manage any underlying conditions, and avoid medications that are harmful to the kidneys.

ANEMIA

Older people with anemia may feel tired and weak all the time, which can affect their general health.

> **Prescription Treatments:** Iron supplements are often used to treat iron-deficiency anemia. For other types, vitamin B12 or folate supplements may be used.
> **Natural Approaches:** A diet high in iron and vitamins (red meat, beans, fortified cereals) can help control and avoid anemia.
> ***Considerations:*** It is important to monitor blood counts and iron levels regularly to determine how well treatment is working and to change doses as needed. If you take iron supplements and have stomach problems, you may need to adjust your food or medications.

Taking care of the health problems that older adults often face takes a multifaceted approach that includes prescription medications, natural and herbal remedies, and practical lifestyle modifications. There are many ways to treat each illness, from arthritis and heart disease to hearing loss and incontinence. The best way to treat each individual is different depending on their specific needs. Some important things to think about are regular monitoring, taking charge of symptoms, and having a strong partnership with healthcare providers to ensure optimal care. By staying informed and involved with their health, older adults can handle the challenges of getting older with grace while maintaining their best quality of life. Using both prescription medications and holistic health practices together can help older adults get healthy in many ways, helping them live full lives despite the complexities of age-related health issues.

11.3 Tailored Medication Choices for the Elderly

When choosing medications for elderly family members, it's important to find a mix between taking care of their health problems and limiting side effects as much as possible to keep their quality of life. I'm here to talk about how to choose medications that are right for older adults based on their specific needs.

Heart Health Considerations:
To reduce high blood pressure, we often look at medications that work well and don't get too much in the way of daily life. Beta-blockers, like metoprolol, work, but they might not always be the best choice for adults because they can make them tired or cause them to have cold hands. Instead, ACE inhibitors or ARBs (like lisinopril or losartan) might be preferable because they can control blood pressure without these drawbacks.

Diabetes Management:
Metformin has been recognized for its effectiveness in managing Type 2 diabetes and for being safe on the kidneys. However, you need to be aware of the side effects of lowering B12 levels, which could have long-term effects. By getting regular check-ups, you can catch this early and ensure that treatment works as well as it can.

Balancing Cholesterol:
Statins are important for controlling high cholesterol, but finding the right dose is important to prevent side effects like muscle pain. Regular liver function tests are also an important part of safe statin treatment because they ensure the drug does its job without putting too much stress on the liver.

Gentle Pain Relief:
Acetaminophen is often preferred for pain relief because it's easy on the stomach. But it's very important to keep an eye on liver health, especially if drinking alcohol often. This ensures that pain relief doesn't come at the expense of liver health.

11.4: The Beers List Explained

Although it's called a list, the Beers List is actually a complete set of guidelines that help healthcare professionals and patients make smart choices about medication use in older adults. This part will summarize the main points of the Beers List and point out common medications that older adults should be careful with, especially those used to treat common diseases in this age group.

Warning About Anticholinergics:
Diphenhydramine and amitriptyline are two examples of these drugs. They may lead to confusion, dry mouth, trouble going to the bathroom, and cause the body to hold on to urine longer. To keep the mind and body in balance, it is good to consider safer alternatives, such as non-drowsy allergy medications like loratadine, cetirizine, or fexofenadine or SSRIs like sertraline for depression.

Caution with Benzodiazepines:
Medications such as lorazepam (Ativan) or diazepam (Valium) are often used to treat nervousness or sleep problems. These make you more likely to fall, get confused, get dizzy, or lose your mental sharpness. Consider gentler options like SSRIs (like sertraline or citalopram), behavioral interventions for anxiety, and non-benzodiazepine sleep aids for insomnia.

Caution on NSAIDs:
Taking NSAIDs like ibuprofen (Advil) or naproxen (Aleve) on a regular basis can cause problems such as Gastrointestinal bleeding, kidney damage, and increased blood pressure. For better pain relief and safety, consider acetaminophen (Tylenol) for pain relief, topical pain treatments for localized pain, or low-dose opioids when you really need them.

Digoxin Dosage:
Digoxin is used to treat heart problems, but older adults need to be careful when taking doses over 0.125 mg/day to prevent toxicity and keep their hearts healthy.

Diabetes Drug Consideration:
Sliding-scale insulin isn't recommended due to the risk of low blood sugar (hypoglycemia). A more stable regimen would involve consistent carbohydrate intake and using long-acting insulin (like Lantus) to manage diabetes wisely.

Antipsychotics:
Antipsychotic drugs, such as haloperidol and olanzapine, come with serious risks, like stroke and memory loss. For managing behavioral issues in older adults with dementia, non-drug methods are preferred. Medications should only be used when necessary and at the lowest amount that works.

> **Hack:** Resources like the American Geriatrics Society and the National Institute on Aging are very helpful and offer a lot of information and advice for people who want to learn more about the Beers List or how to take medications safely as an older adult.

Sedative-hypnotics
These include medications like zolpidem, which come with big risks like being sleepy during the day, getting confused, and making you more likely to fall. Sleep hygiene practices, melatonin, or short-term use of non-sedating medications should be considered first.

When it comes to managing medications for elderly adults, the Beers List is a great guide for choosing safer medications. By learning and following the rules in the Beers List, we can lower the risks of medication use in older adults while also improving their quality of life and health. To make sure that their medication plans are safe and successful, they need to be carefully chosen, reviewed regularly, and closely watched.

11.5: Opioids and Benzodiazepines

As we get older, our bodies don't handle medications as well as they used to, making it easier for us to feel the effects and side effects more strongly. Benzodiazepines, which are used to treat nervousness and insomnia, and opioids, which are strong painkillers, are two types of drugs that are especially likely to cause this. I'm here to help you understand how these medicines work, why they might not be safe for older people, and the right way to take them.

Understanding Opioids

Opioids, which include oxycodone, hydrocodone, and morphine, are strong painkillers that are often recommended for a wide range of conditions, such as after surgery or giving birth. But these drugs can be hard for older people. They can make you sleepy, sluggish, sick, and even slow down your breathing. People who use them are also more likely to become dependent on them and are more likely to fall, which can cause major injuries.

Understanding Benzodiazepines

People often get benzodiazepines, such as diazepam (Valium), lorazepam (Ativan), and alprazolam (Xanax), to help with nervousness, muscle spasms, and insomnia. However, they can be problematic for older adults because they can cause them to be more forgetful, feel dizzy, and be more likely to fall. These medications should only be used for a short time, and other methods should be considered first if possible.

Combining Opioids and Benzodiazepines: Extra Caution Needed

When it comes to medications, opioids and benzodiazepines are two powerful medications. When used together, they can be dangerous, so be extra careful. This is because both opioids and benzodiazepines have a calming effect on the body and can slow down vital functions such as breathing. When taken in combination, these effects are multiplied, increasing the risks of slowed breathing, extreme drowsiness, or even life-threatening situations. This combination can also increase the likelihood of accidents, such as falls, which are particularly dangerous for older adults.

TIPS FOR SAFE USE OF COMBINATION
OPIOIDS AND BENZODIAZEPINES

Avoid Taking Together:
If you need to take both medications together, try not to do so at the same time. Taking them at different times, usually at least 4 to 6 hours apart, can help lower the risk of side effects. The number of hours between doses will depend on the medications, so check with your doctor to make sure you know how long you need to wait based on the medications you take.

Look into other options:
If possible, talk to your doctor about other treatments that might work instead of opioids and benzodiazepines instead to meet your needs. Alternative medications or treatments may work just as well and have fewer side effects.

Start Low, Go Slow:
Let's say we have to take both opioids and benzodiazepines together. In that case, the key is to start with the smallest amounts possible and only raise them if needed. This approach will help lower the risk of side effects that you don't want.

Pay Attention to How You Feel:
If you're taking both, it's important to monitor your symptoms and tell your doctor or pharmacist right away about any that are bothering you. Key signs to watch for are extreme drowsiness, having a hard time waking up, slow or shallow breathing, or confusion.

Educate Yourself and Others:
Having a plan and knowing the signs of an overdose can save lives. Make sure you and the people around you know what to do in this situation.

Review Regularly

It's important to check in with your doctor often to see if you still need to be taking any of your medications. Changes in your condition might allow for a lower dosage or stopping one or both of the medications. The decision to use opioids and benzodiazepines in the elderly should never be taken lightly, especially in combination. While they can be helpful, they come with risks, especially for the elderly. By managing these medications carefully, staying in close contact with your healthcare providers, and considering non-drug treatments, you can lessen these risks and still get relief from pain, anxiety, or sleep issues.

SAFEGUARDING WITH NARCAN WHEN COMBINING OPIOIDS AND BENZODIAZEPINES

If you are ever in a situation where an opioid overdose has occurred, Narcan (naloxone) is a lifesaving tool. Narcan is an opioid antagonist, meaning it can quickly reverse the effects of opioid overdose, potentially saving lives. Narcan can act within minutes to reverse the effects of opioid overdose. It is available as a nasal spray, making it easy to use, even for those without medical training. It's important to still call 911 immediately after using it since additional medical help might be needed.

Due to the increase in opioid-related overdoses, many states have made Narcan more accessible to the public. You can often obtain it from pharmacies without a prescription, and some insurance plans may cover it.

Narcan is a very important safety net that can be used in the event of an opioid overdose. You can lower the risks of these medications by keeping an eye out for signs of overdose, keeping Narcan on hand in case of an emergency, and making sure you and everyone around you know how to use it.

Medication management for the elderly includes knowing their specific medical needs, recognizing the most common illnesses they have, and choosing appropriate medications to treat them. Tailored medication choices, supported by tools like the Beers List, lead to safer prescribing, lowering risks and improving outcomes for patients. To find the right mix between effectiveness and safety, extra care needs to be taken when managing medications with higher risk profiles, like opioids and benzodiazepines. The goal is to optimize the quality of life for older adults by giving them educated, individualized, and compassionate medication management. This shows how important it is to take a cautious and comprehensive approach when caring for the elderly.

FURTHER READING FOR CHAPTER 11:
ELDERLY MEDICATION MANAGEMENT

American Geriatrics Society (AGS)
For guidance on managing medications for the elderly and the Beers List, visit the American Geriatrics Society.
Available at: www.americangeriatrics.org.

National Institute on Aging (NIA)
Explore detailed information on treatments for common ailments in the elderly and general health management tips from the National Institute on Aging.
Available at: www.nia.nih.gov.

Geriatric Medicine Research
For research and insights into tailored medication choices for the elderly, Geriatric Medicine Research provides a range of resources and study findings.
Available at: www.geriatric.theclinics.com.

Substance Abuse and Mental Health Services Administration (SAMHSA)
Learn about the use and management of opioids and benzodiazepines in the elderly, including safety guidelines and risk factors, through SAMHSA.
Available at: www.samhsa.gov.

American Society of Consultant Pharmacists (ASCP)
For information on medication management in older adults, particularly in the context of complex health issues, visit the American Society of Consultant Pharmacists.
Available at: www.ascp.com

FOR MORE INFORMATION
ON SPECIFIC MEDICAL CONDITIONS,
HERE ARE ADDITIONAL RESOURCES

American Heart Association (AHA)
For information on heart health and blood pressure management, visit the American Heart Association.
Available at: www.heart.org.

American Diabetes Association (ADA)
For resources on diabetes management and treatments, visit the American Diabetes Association.
Available at: www.diabetes.org.

National Kidney Foundation (NKF)
For information on kidney health and chronic kidney disease management, visit the National Kidney Foundation.
Available at: www.kidney.org.

Arthritis Foundation
Offers detailed information on managing arthritis, including medication options and lifestyle tips. Visit the Arthritis Foundation.
Available at: www.arthritis.org.

National Institutes of Health – National Heart, Lung, and Blood Institute (NHLBI)
For comprehensive information on managing cardiovascular and respiratory diseases, visit the National Heart, Lung, and Blood Institute.
Available at: www.nhlbi.nih.gov.

Alzheimer's Association
For resources on managing Alzheimer's disease and dementia, visit the Alzheimer's Association.
Available at: www.alz.org.

American Gastroenterological Association (AGA)
For information on gastrointestinal issues and management strategies, visit the American Gastroenterological Association.
Available at: www.gastro.org.

American Academy of Ophthalmology (AAO)
For insights into eye health, including age-related macular degeneration and glaucoma management, visit the American Academy of Ophthalmology.
Available at: www.aao.org.

CHAPTER 12:
MEDICATIONS DURING PREGNANCY AND NURSING

Becoming pregnant or nursing changes how you handle your medications in important ways. Everything you take and do is more important than ever. In this chapter, you'll learn about the medications that are safe and recommended to take during this special time. I'll help you understand the different types of pregnancy categories as well as help you pick out prenatal supplements that are good for your health and the health of your baby. To make informed decisions without putting your baby's safety at risk, we'll also talk about common ailments experienced during pregnancy and the treatment options that are recommended, safe, and effective. There are special considerations that are important for both pregnant and nursing mothers. I'll go over them carefully and completely so you can feel confident and informed.

12.1: Pregnancy Category Insights

It can be hard to find your way around medications while you are pregnant or nursing. I'm here to help you and make sure you and your baby stay healthy. Here is a breakdown of how drugs are grouped during pregnancy. This will help you understand what is safe and what you should avoid.

Category A:
These are the recommended medications to take while you're pregnant. They've been studied carefully and don't pose any risks to your baby. This

group includes prenatal vitamins, which are very important for your baby's growth and provide important nutrients.

Category B:
These medications are like cautious friends and are generally considered safe. Studies haven't shown that they harm animals, but there aren't comprehensive human studies. Acetaminophen (Tylenol) is part of this category. It's often used to treat pain and has not been shown to harm the unborn child.

Category C:
We need to be careful here. Animal tests have shown that these medications may have some risks, but we might still use them if the benefits are greater than the risks. An example from this category is spironolactone (Aldactone), a water pill used to treat edema, and heart conditions. Some cold and cough medications, like guaifenesin (Mucinex) and Dextromethorphan (Robitussin), are also in this group.

Category D:
These medications come with a warning label. There is proof that they may be bad for your baby, but in some cases, their benefits might still be greater than the risks. Certain medications for seizures fit here; they're not ideal, but sometimes they're needed.

Category X:
Medications in this class should never be taken. The risks are greater than the rewards due to the high risk of causing serious birth defects. Isotretinoin (Accutane), a medication used for severe acne, belongs in this class.

For women who are nursing, the most important thing is to know if the medication gets into the breast milk. Some, like the decongestant pseudoephedrine, may make it harder to breastfeed due to its effects on reducing milk supply, so it's advisable to stay away while nursing.

It's important to weigh the pros and cons and consult your healthcare provider before starting or stopping any medications. For minor ailments, try treatments that don't involve taking medications first. Simple changes to your lifestyle or home remedies can be effective and safer. Being aware of how to take medications during these special times safely can help protect both you and your baby.

12.2: Prenatal Vitamin Guide

Prenatals are not just some old multivitamin; think of them as your pregnancy super team. They are packed with goodies like folic acid, iron, calcium, and DHA, which are all important for keeping you and your baby healthy as they grow. Allow me to explain why they're so great:

Folic Acid:
This vitamin is very important because it helps prevent dangerous problems, like neural tube defects, in babies from the start. Aim for 400 to 600 micrograms every day

Iron:
It's important because it helps you and your baby get the oxygen you need and keeps your energy up.

Calcium:
This is good for your baby's bones and teeth. It also keeps your muscles, nerves, and blood circulation in tip-top shape, so you're not giving up your bone strength while your baby grows.

DHA:
DHA is an Omega-3 that is important for your baby's brain and eye development. Adding DHA to your daily routine is like giving your baby a head start on their development.

No doubt, prenatal vitamins are important—they're your nutrition power-up during pregnancy. They have your back (and your baby's, too) and will make sure you both get the support you need every step of the way. Think of them as something you do every day, like drinking coffee in the morning, but with a whole lot of benefits for you and your bump.

12.3: Safe Treatments for Common Ailments

Becoming a mother comes with its own set of challenges, such as figuring out how to deal with the common ailments that come with pregnancy and breastfeeding. From the waves of morning sickness to the ripples of changes after giving birth, it's important to know about these conditions and how to treat them safely. This part goes over the 20 most common health problems that pregnant and nursing moms have, showing you how to find safe and effective solutions.

MORNING SICKNESS

During the first few months of pregnancy, morning sickness is common and can range from mild nausea to serious vomiting.

> **Dietary Adjustments:** Eating small meals more often, snacking on bland foods like crackers, or eating plain rice can help.
> **Ginger:** Ginger tea or ginger candies are natural remedies that can help with nausea.
> **Medications:** Vitamin B6 and doxylamine are both safe and often recommended. If the nausea is severe, your healthcare provider might prescribe an anti-nausea medication called ondansetron.
> ***Considerations:*** Stay hydrated and avoid triggers that cause nausea, like strong odors. If morning sickness makes it hard to do normal daily things or causes significant weight loss, see a doctor.

HEARTBURN AND INDIGESTION

Hormonal changes and the pressure of the growing uterus on the gut can cause heartburn and indigestion in many pregnant women.

> **Lifestyle Modifications:** Eating smaller meals more often and staying away from acidic and spicy foods can help reduce symptoms.
> **Antacids:** Calcium carbonate and other over-the-counter antacids can reduce stomach acid and provide relief.

Medications: If you have persistent heartburn, your doctor may suggest taking an H2 blocker such as famotidine (Pepcid) or a proton pump inhibitor like pantoprazole and omeprazole. Both are available as prescription medications or may be purchased over the counter.
Considerations: Avoid lying down right after eating, and raise the head of the bed to help prevent heartburn or indigestion from happening at night.

FATIGUE

Hormonal changes and the physical demands of supporting a growing baby can make pregnant women feel tired.

Rest: Getting enough sleep and taking short naps can help.
Nutrition: A balanced diet rich in iron and proteins can give you more energy.
Mild Exercise: Walking or practicing prenatal yoga can give you more energy and can also improve sleep.
Considerations: The key is finding a good balance between activity and rest. If you're tired and have other symptoms, like shortness of breath or heart palpitations, consult a healthcare provider. Checking for iron deficiency would be helpful, since it is a common cause of fatigue in pregnancy.

BACK PAIN

Being pregnant can cause back pain because of the extra weight, changes in posture, and the way hormones affect joints and tendons.

Exercise: Prenatal yoga and stretches can help strengthen the back and ease pain.
Supportive Gear: Back pain can be relieved by using Maternity belts or comfortable shoes.
Therapies: Therapies like physiotherapy, acupuncture, or massage may help as long as you follow your doctor's advice.

Considerations: keep your back straight, don't lift big things, and use heat or cold packs to ease pain.

CONSTIPATION

The digestive system slows down during pregnancy due to changes in hormones, causing constipation.

Dietary Fiber: Eating foods with high fiber content, such as vegetables and whole grains, can help prevent constipation.
Hydration: It's important to drink a lot of water to make going to the bathroom easier.
Stool Softeners: Mild laxatives such as MiraLax or stool softeners like docusate are usually safe to use while pregnant, but you should talk to your doctor first.
Considerations: Regular physical activity can also help promote healthy digestive function. If constipation lasts for a long time, you should see a doctor for safe and effective treatment.

GESTATIONAL DIABETES

This happens when blood sugar levels are high during pregnancy and can be harmful to both the mother and the baby.

Exercise and Diet: Regular exercise and a diet low in simple sugars can help keep blood sugar levels in check.
Monitoring Blood Sugar: Checking blood sugar often lets you make changes to your food or medications at the right time to keep glucose levels under control.
Insulin therapy: Insulin injections may be needed if food and exercise are not enough to keep blood sugar levels under control.
Metformin: This medication helps control gestational diabetes by improving the body's response to insulin and lowering glucose production in the liver.

Considerations: It's important to carefully control gestational diabetes to prevent complications like preterm birth and others in the newborn. Monitoring should continue after giving birth because gestational diabetes can make it more likely to develop type 2 diabetes later in life.

PREECLAMPSIA

Preeclampsia is characterized by high blood pressure as well as signs of damage to other organs, such as the kidneys or liver.

> **Regular Monitoring:** It's important to keep a close eye on blood pressure, as well as liver and kidney function.
> **Medications:** To control blood pressure, antihypertensive drugs such as labetalol or nifedipine may be given.
> **Delivery:** In serious situations, an early delivery may be suggested to prevent major problems for the mother and baby.
> ***Considerations:*** To ensure the safety of both mother and child, people with preeclampsia need to see their doctor often for pregnancy checkups and may need bed rest.

INSOMNIA

Hormonal changes, physical pain, or stress can make it hard for many pregnant women to sleep.

> **Sleep Hygiene:** Setting up a routine at night and making the sleeping area comfortable can improve sleep quality.
> **Relaxation Techniques:** Activities like prenatal yoga, meditation, or light stretching can promote better sleep.
> **Medications:** If needed, doctors may suggest sleep aids such as doxylamine, which are safe for pregnant women, unlike other sleep aids. However, they should only be used when necessary. Diphenhydramine (Benadryl) is sometimes used, but its safety is not fully confirmed.
> ***Considerations:*** Don't drink coffee or eat big meals right before bed; use pillows to support your body, and find a comfortable sleeping position.

VARICOSE VEINS

Varicose veins can happen in the legs because of the extra blood and higher blood pressure that come with pregnancy.

> **Compression Stockings:** These relieve the pressure in the veins and can help improve blood flow throughout the legs.
> **Elevating the Legs:** Keeping your legs raised above your heart level can lower blood pressure and help with vein pressure and swelling.
> **Exercise:** Walking and other low-impact exercises can help with circulation and lessen your symptoms.
> ***Considerations:*** To reduce pressure on the veins, avoid sitting or standing for too long and maintain a healthy weight.

HEMORRHOIDS

Because of the pressure from the growing uterus and more blood flow, pregnancy makes getting hemorrhoids more likely.

> **Dietary Fiber:** Eating fiber-rich foods can help prevent constipation and make going to the bathroom easier.
> **Hydration:** Drinking plenty of water also makes stools softer, which makes hemorrhoids less painful.
> **Topical treatments:** Creams and ointments, such as Preparation H, which are available over the counter, can help with pain and swelling.
> ***Considerations:*** Do not strain when going to the bathroom, and see a doctor if hemorrhoids cause significant pain or bleeding.

URINARY TRACT INFECTIONS (UTIS)

Because of changes in the body, pregnancy often causes UTIs. Getting immediate treatment is important to prevent complications.

> **Antibiotics:** Certain antibiotics, like amoxicillin or nitrofurantoin, are usually recommended to treat UTIs and are safe for pregnant women.

Hydration: Drinking more water helps get rid of bacteria in the urinary system.
Cranberry Juice: Cranberry juice has been known to help lower the chance of UTIs by stopping bacteria from sticking to the bladder walls.
Considerations: To make sure the infection is completely gone, it's important to take all of the medications as prescribed. While pregnant, it may be best to get checked for UTIs on a regular basis.

YEAST INFECTIONS

Due to having more estrogen in the body while pregnant, the risk of getting a vaginal yeast infection is higher.

Antifungal Creams or Suppositories: Miconazole or clotrimazole are examples of safe and useful products that can be used during pregnancy.
Probiotics: Eating foods like yogurt that are high in probiotics can help keep your vaginal flora healthy.
Good Hygiene: Keeping the vaginal area dry and clean can help prevent the growth of yeast.
Considerations: If you are pregnant, don't use oral antifungal treatments on your own. Instead, talk to your doctor about the right treatment. Probiotics should be taken at least 2 to 3 hours after the antibiotic dose so that the antibiotic won't immediately kill the beneficial bacteria in the probiotics.

EDEMA (SWELLING)

People who are pregnant often have swollen feet and ankles due to increased body fluids and blood flow during pregnancy.

Elevation Keeping the feet elevated can help lessen swelling.
Compression stockings: These can help get more blood flowing and help the body keep less water in the legs.
Exercise: Walking or swimming are gentle exercises that can help reduce swelling by getting the blood flowing.

Considerations: Mild edema is normal, but sudden or serious swelling could be a sign of preeclampsia and needs to be checked out right away by a healthcare provider.

STRETCH MARKS

These are common during pregnancy because the skin stretches as the baby grows. They happen more often with significant weight gain in a short period instead of gradual and slow.

> **Moisturizers and Oils:** Products with cocoa butter, vitamin E, or hyaluronic acid can help keep the skin soft and lessen the appearance of stretch marks.
> **Hydration:** Keeping your body hydrated helps the skin stay elastic.
> **Balanced Diet:** Eating foods rich in vitamins and minerals is good for skin health and can help prevent severe stretch marks.
> ***Considerations:*** How well topical treatments works in preventing stretch marks is not strongly supported by evidence. Many methods claim to get rid of stretch marks, but how well they work can vary. It might also help to accept these changes as normal parts of being pregnant. Genetics also play a role, as some are more prone to developing them than others.

BREAST PAIN AND CHANGES

Changes in hormones during pregnancy and nursing can make breasts sore and cause them to get bigger.

> **Supportive Bras:** A supportive bra that fits well can help with the discomfort.
> **Warm or Cold Compresses:** Applying heat or cold on an area can help with pain and swelling.
> **Pain Relief:** Over-the-counter pain medications like acetaminophen (Tylenol), but you should talk to your healthcare provider before taking any medications while pregnant or nursing.

Considerations: Breast pain and size changes in the breasts are usually normal, but it's important to keep an eye out for any strange symptoms, like lumps or pain that won't go away, and talk to your healthcare provider about them.

LEG CRAMPS

People who are pregnant often have leg cramps, which are sudden, painful muscle twitches. This is especially true in the second and third trimesters.

Stretching Exercises: Stretching the calm muscles before bed can help prevent leg cramps.
Magnesium Supplements: With your doctor's approval, taking magnesium supplements can also help with leg cramps.
Staying Hydrated: Being well hydrated helps muscles work properly and can also help prevent leg cramps.
Considerations: Though leg cramps are generally not dangerous if they last for a long time or are very painful, you should see a doctor. The pain might be something more serious, such as deep vein thrombosis or DVT, which would need to be ruled out by your healthcare provider. If you do experience a leg cramp, gently massaging the legs can help the leg cramp subside.

NASAL PROBLEMS

Pregnancy rhinitis, often experienced as nasal congestion or frequent nosebleeds, occurs because of the increased blood volume during pregnancy.

Saline Nasal Sprays: These are a safe and effective way to clear up stuffy noses.
Humidifiers: Having a humidifier nearby can keep the nasal passages moist and relieve discomfort.
Avoiding Irritants: To help reduce nasal problems, stay away from smoke and other irritants.
Considerations: During pregnancy, avoid using over-the-counter decongestants unless specifically advised by your healthcare provider.

NASAL CONGESTION

When you're pregnant, your nasal passages can get swollen, which can make it hard to breathe.

> **Steam Treatment:** Taking deep breaths of steam from a vaporizer, a hot shower, or over a bowl of hot water can help clear the nose.
> **Elevated Sleeping Position:** Sleeping with an extra pillow under your head can help with nighttime congestion.
> **Nasal Strips:** These can be put on the nose at night to help open the nasal passages and make breathing easier.
> ***Considerations:*** Most doctors don't suggest over-the-counter nasal decongestants for pregnant women, so natural and physical ways to clear up congestion are better options.

ANEMIA

Anemia, especially iron deficiency anemia, is common during pregnancy and can cause fatigue and other symptoms.

> **Iron supplements:** These are often recommended to boost iron levels, but they should only be taken under the supervision of a doctor because they can cause side effects like constipation.
> **Dietary Sources of Iron:** You can also eat foods with high iron content, such as leafy greens, beans, and lean meats.
> **Vitamin C:** This vitamin, when eaten with iron-rich foods, helps the body absorb iron better.
> ***Considerations:*** Regular blood tests are recommended to monitor iron levels, and treatment should be adjusted to prevent too-high iron levels, which can be harmful.

MOOD SWINGS AND MENTAL HEALTH ISSUES

Hormonal changes can affect mood, which increases the potential to experience stress, anxiety, and sadness during and after giving birth.

Counseling and Support Groups: Attending therapy can provide significant relief and support.

Mindfulness and Relaxation Techniques: Practicing yoga, meditation, and deep breathing are all good ways to improve mental health and well-being.

Medications: Antidepressants such as sertraline (Zoloft) or anxiety medications can be helpful. But only with strict medical supervision.

Considerations: It's very important to deal with mental health problems and get help from a professional immediately. Mental health problems that aren't treated can affect both the mother and the baby.

During pregnancy and nursing, there are unique health challenges that require well-informed decisions. This guide to common ailments shows a range of choices, from conventional medication to natural remedies, all of which are based on the idea of being safe and effective. It's important to use a comprehensive approach that includes lifestyle modifications and preventative care. Women who are pregnant or nursing can take charge of their health and make sure that they and their children are healthy and happy by working together with doctors and nurses and choosing treatments carefully.

> **Hack:** Fenugreek is a popular herb for boosting milk supply, but it's not for everyone. If you have a sensitive stomach or if you notice that it directly upsets your or your baby's stomach, you might need to skip it.

12.4: Considerations for Pregnant and Nursing Women

Here are some special considerations to remember if you are pregnant or nursing. It's a short list, but it's important to stay healthy while pregnant and nursing.

FOR BREASTFEEDING MOMS

Coffee:
One or two small cups a day is fine, so it doesn't make the baby jittery or keep them from sleeping.

Alcohol:
It's best not to take any, but if you do drink, it's best not to nurse for two to three hours after each drink. Waiting will give your body time to break down the alcohol.

CAUTION WITH
COMMON MEDICATIONS

Cold and Allergy Medications:
Pseudoephedrine (Sudafed) can lower milk production. Better alternatives are phenylephrine (Sudafed PE) or diphenhydramine (Benadryl). Always consult with your healthcare provider first.

Certain Antibiotics:
Most are safe, but certain kinds, like tetracyclines, can affect the baby's teeth and bone growth.

NSAIDs:
It is better to avoid NSAIDS like ibuprofen (Advil) and naproxen (Aleve).. They affect the baby's kidneys and blood circulation, especially when taken in the third trimester.

Certain Medications for Blood Pressure:
ACE Inhibitors like lisinopril can cause serious harm to the developing baby. Talk to your healthcare provider if you are taking this medication.

Opioids:
Codeine and other opioids, such as hydrocodone or oxycodone, are typically not recommended because they can affect your baby's breathing.

HERBAL REMEDIES:
NATURAL DOESN'T ALWAYS MEAN SAFE

Echinacea:
Although echinacea is often used to treat colds, its safety during pregnancy and nursing hasn't been studied much. Once you've talked to your doctor, it's best to stick with vitamin C and zinc tablets to keep your immune system strong.

St. John's Wort:
It is used for mild depression, but it can interact with many other medications. Its effects on babies whose mothers are feeding them are not fully known. Always discuss with your doctor before use.

Wrapping it all up...

When it comes to managing your health during pregnancy and while breastfeeding, the safest approach is always to consult with your healthcare provider first before taking any medications, including OTC or herbal treatments; they can help weigh the risks and benefits, making sure that you and your baby are both healthy and safe. Remember that this information is just a starting point. Your OB/GYN or pediatrician is the best resource to get advice that is specific to your health needs.

> **Hack:** If you want to know exactly what is safe and what isn't, the American Pregnancy Association and LactMed databases are like your own personal library of knowledge. They are always up-to-date and reliable.

FURTHER READING FOR CHAPTER 12:
MEDICATIONS DURING PREGNANCY AND NURSING

American College of Obstetricians and Gynecologists (ACOG)
For expert guidelines on medication use during pregnancy and lactation, including insights into pregnancy categories, visit the American College of Obstetricians and Gynecologists.
Available at: www.acog.org.

March of Dimes
Explore comprehensive resources on prenatal vitamins and safe treatments for common ailments during pregnancy provided by the March of Dimes.
Available at: www.marchofdimes.org.

La Leche League International
Gain insights into medication considerations for nursing mothers, including safe practices and recommendations, from La Leche League International.
Available at: www.llli.org.

American Pregnancy Association
For comprehensive guidance on managing pregnancy-related health conditions, visit the American Pregnancy Association.
Available at: www.americanpregnancy.org.

Centers for Disease Control and Prevention (CDC)
For information on pregnancy health and safety tips, consult the Centers for Disease Control and Prevention.
Available at: www.cdc.gov/pregnancy.

March of Dimes
For resources and support on pregnancy, including management of common conditions, refer to the March of Dimes.
Available at: www.marchofdimes.org.

U.S. Food and Drug Administration (FDA)
For details on medication safety during pregnancy, visit the U.S. Food and Drug Administration.
Available at: www.fda.gov.

Mayo Clinic
For expert health advice on pregnancy and managing pregnancy symptoms, see the Mayo Clinic's resources.
Available at: www.mayoclinic.org/healthy-lifestyle/pregnancy-week-by-week.

CHAPTER 13:
SAFE MEDICATION PRACTICES

Take a step toward better health and well-being by learning how to handle medications safely. I'm here to help you understand the most important parts of medication safety. I'll cover how important it is to read and understand medication labels, as well as how important it is to double-check everything, from the drug's name to its expiration date. I'll help you avoid common mistakes of underdosing or overdosing by talking about dose and timing and why accuracy is not just a nice thing to do but a must. Additionally, we'll talk about the dangerous aspects of sharing medications and stress why your prescription should remain yours alone. In the case of medication recalls, I'll show you how to stay safe by staying proactive. Join me in breaking down the rules of safe medication practices in this chapter.

13.1: Understanding Safe Practices

READ AND UNDERSTAND

For safe and effective use, each medication comes with its own set of directions and information. When you pick up a medication, you'll find a leaflet inside the packaging. This leaflet is your mini-guidebook. It tells you about usual side effects, things you should know, and the best way to take your medication.

During your medication pick-up, the pharmacist will highlight some of these points to make sure you understand how to take the medication(s) properly. They'll cover how much and how often you should take your medication, what to do if you miss a dose, and any changes you may need to make to your lifestyle.

These leaflets also include special considerations. Here are some common examples you might see if you decide to crack open and read those mini-guidebooks:

Drug interactions:
Certain medications or over-the-counter supplements can affect how your medications work when taken together. Always let your doctor and pharmacist know about all the medications you are taking.

Lifestyle Factors:
What you eat, how much you exercise, and even how you sleep can affect how well your medication works. For example, some medications may make you more sensitive to sunlight, and others may make you sick when you eat certain foods.

Alcohol Interaction:
Having alcohol with medications like metronidazole (Flagyl), commonly used for certain bacterial and parasitic infections, can cause severe reactions like nausea and vomiting even up to several days after stopping the antibiotic.

Remember, the goal here is to understand the 'why.' For that reason, if you ever don't understand something on a medication label or leaflet, or if you want to know how to start taking a new medication, talk to your pharmacist or doctor.

DOUBLE-CHECK EVERY DETAIL

If you're careful, you can catch mistakes before they happen. Whenever you get medication, even if it is a refill, take a moment to review it and watch for the following:

Verify Dose and Strength:
If you've recently seen or talked to your doctor, the dose or strength of your medications may have changed. Often, these changes are made to fine-tune your treatment based on how you're acting or to help you better handle side effects. As an example, if you were taking 20 mg of lisinopril for high blood pressure and it wasn't quite lowering it to the right level, your doctor might raise the amount to 40 mg. Make sure that the medication you get now fits these changes.

Check for Medication Switches:
Sometimes, your doctor may switch you to an alternative medication to replace the one you were taking before. One reason for this could be that the medication doesn't work, has side effects, or isn't covered by insurance. For example, if you were taking atorvastatin to lower your cholesterol, your doctor may switch you to simvastatin depending on how your body reacts or if your insurance plan changes. The medication you pick up must reflect this switch.

> **Hack:** Unless your doctor's office contacts your pharmacy, they won't be aware of these changes in dose, medication, or discontinuations, so make sure to communicate with the pharmacy to avoid picking up a medication you are no longer taking. It might also help to bring an updated list to the pharmacy and have them check it against your active medications in the pharmacy system.

Confirm Continuation or Discontinuation:
Your doctor may have told you to stop taking a medication, but your pharmacy wasn't told. If you don't pay attention, you might keep taking a medication that isn't part of your treatment plan anymore. For example, if metformin was stopped because it caused stomach problems, but you are still getting it because the pharmacy wasn't updated, this could cause you unnecessary discomfort or confusion.

Check for Alternative Manufacturers:
If you pick up your medication and notice that it doesn't look like the others you've seen, there's a good reason for that, and you shouldn't worry about it. When medications come from different manufacturers, they may

look different in terms of color, shape, or size. This often happens because pharmacies might switch suppliers based on availability or cost. The medication will still work just as well because it has the same active ingredient, which is what makes it work as a treatment. However, the inactive ingredients, which are things like fillers or dyes that don't change how the medication works, can be different. These differences are only for looks; they don't affect how well or how safe the medications are. If your medication looks different, you should always talk to your pharmacist about it. They'll make sure it's the right medication, giving you peace of mind.

Always read the labels on your medications before leaving the pharmacy. Compare the name of the drug, the amount to be taken, and the directions with what your doctor told you. If something seems off or you're not sure, don't be afraid to ask your pharmacist to check it again for you. We can check it against the prescription your doctor gave us.

> **Hack:** The label on your medication bottle describes how the medication should look, including shape, colors, and markings. If the name matches the medication you are taking and the description on the bottle matches the pill inside, then you have the correct medication. If you are still unsure, you can always double-check by asking your local pharmacist.

Always remember that your health and safety come first. By checking your medications twice, you are protecting yourself from potential errors and ensuring that your treatment continues properly.

13.2: Dosage and Timing Importance

Understanding how and when to take your medication isn't just medical advice; it's a strategy for getting the most out of your prescriptions. Each medication or treatment comes with a plan for getting the most out of it while avoiding side effects that you don't want.

Why timing is important

Think of medications like levothyroxine (Synthroid), which helps people with thyroid problems. It works best on an empty stomach, 30 to 60 minutes before breakfast. This little trick will make sure that your body absorbs it fully. If you do it too close to a meal, on the other hand, it might not work as well, leaving your thyroid playing catch-up.

Consistency Wins the Race

Then there are medications like warfarin that thin the blood. When you take it is just as important as how much you take it. Sticking to a routine helps keep your blood perfectly balanced, avoiding clots or the opposite—bleeding risks. Diabetics face a similar need for insulin or sugar-managing meds. To keep blood sugar from going up and down like a roller coaster, they need to take medications or inject insulin at regular times.

How to Nail Dosage and Timing

Sticking to regular medication schedules, especially if you are taking a lot of different kinds, can seem daunting. To keep things on track, here are some tips:

Pill Organizers and Apps

Pillboxes and even smart apps can help you remember what, when, and how much to take. Using alarms on your smartphone is great for more than just waking you up or reminding you to call Mom. They're also great for reminding you to take your medicine.

Routines are helpful

If you connect your medication to daily activities, like meal times for "take with food" medications or sleep for evening doses, you can easily fit them into your day. One example is that taking your statins at night might work perfectly with your body's cholesterol workshop.

If you don't follow the directions for dosage and timing, your medications may not work as well, which could cause health problems. In the case of antibiotics, you could also be adding to the growing worry of antibiotic resistance. So, keep it consistent, and when in doubt, your pharmacist is always here.

13.3: Risks of Medication Sharing

Sharing medicine with someone in a pinch might seem safe or even helpful, but there are serious risks that you should be aware of. People are given medications after a full evaluation of their health condition, which includes their medical history, present health condition, and specific treatment needs.

Risk of Unchecked Drug Interactions:
When medications are shared, the important step of having the medication checked for possible drug interactions is skipped. For instance, giving someone else a prescription painkiller that works well for you could put their health at great risk if they are also taking other drugs that combine badly with it.

Side Effects and Adverse Reactions:
All medications have the potential for side effects, which are carefully thought through when they are prescribed. A medication that causes minimal side effects for you might cause severe adverse reactions in someone else due to differences in health conditions, allergies, or sensitivities. For example, a popular beta-blocker used to treat high blood pressure could cause dangerous drops in blood pressure in someone whose health or medications have not been checked for the addition of the medication.

Incorrect Dosage and Usage:
Each medication comes with specific dosage directions that are made to fit the needs of the patient. When people share medications, the person who gets them often takes a dose that hasn't been adjusted for their treatment. This can lead to underdosing, overdosing, or the wrong use of the medication. This not only makes the medication less effective, but it could also lead to dangerous health outcomes.

By following these guidelines and examples, you'll ensure your medications work as intended, from the first dose to the last. Remember, if you're not sure, your pharmacist is your go-to resource. They can give you information that is specific to your needs and medications.

13.4: Medication Recall Procedures

Let's talk about something really important—medication recalls. As a patient, I want to make sure you know what to do if a medication you are taking is recalled. Even though it doesn't happen often, it's important to know what to do in case it does.

Why Do Medications Get Recalled?
First, why would a medication be recalled? Several reasons can lead to recalls, such as contamination, wrong labels or dose information, or discovering harmful side effects. It's all about keeping you safe from potential harm.

What Should You Do If Your Medication Is Called Back?
Don't worry. It can be stressful to find out that the medication you are taking has been recalled, but it's important to keep calm. When a drug is recalled, you don't always have to stop taking it right away. The problem might not always be with the safety of the drug itself but with how it is packaged or how stable it is over time.

> **Hack:** You can check the FDA's page on recalls at www.fda.gov/safety/recalls-market-withdrawals-safety-alerts or call your local pharmacy.

Check the Specifics:
If you hear that a medication you're taking is being recalled, the first thing you should do is make sure you understand what is being recalled. In recalls, the batch number, expiration dates, and other identifiers are often given.

Talk to a Healthcare Professional:
Talk to your doctor or pharmacist before you decide what to do. They can tell you if you should stop taking the medication right away or if it's safer to keep taking it until an option is available.

Follow the Instructions for Returning the Medication:
If the medication is part of a recall and needs to be sent back, follow the instructions. These are typically outlined on a recall letter or posted on the website. This could mean taking the medication back to your pharmacy or following specific disposal guidelines.

Secure a Replacement:
If you need to, work with your doctor to find a good replacement or an alternative medication. If you have a chronic condition, you should never stop or change your medication without first talking to a healthcare provider.

HOW TO KNOW ABOUT PRESCRIPTION RECALLS AND GET READY FOR THEM

Part of taking good care of your health is staying up to date on drug recalls. Here are some more things you can do to keep moving forward:

Sign up for alerts:
Many health agencies and pharmacies have systems that send out recall alerts. You can get a heads-up as soon as a recall is announced if you sign up.

Keep Your Medication List Up-To-Date:
Keeping an up-to-date list of your medications, including dosages and the doctors who prescribed them, helps in managing a recall smoothly.

Check Expiration Dates and Batch Numbers:
Check the expiration dates and batch numbers of your medications regularly, especially if you have long-term prescriptions. If you don't have the original bottle, you can contact your pharmacy to double-check the expiration dates and batch numbers they used for you against a current recall.

Remember that medication recalls are about preventing harm and ensuring that the treatments you rely on are safe and effective.

FURTHER READING FOR CHAPTER 13:
SAFE MEDICATION PRACTICES

Institute for Safe Medication Practices (ISMP)
For a comprehensive guide on understanding safe medication practices and detailed information on avoiding common medication errors, visit the Institute for Safe Medication Practices.
Available at: www.ismp.org.

U.S. Food and Drug Administration (FDA)
Learn about the importance of dosage and timing, and explore resources on medication recall procedures from the U.S. Food and Drug Administration.
Available at: www.fda.gov.

Centers for Disease Control and Prevention (CDC)
Discover guidelines and educational resources about the risks of medication sharing, including the potential health implications, provided by the CDC.
Available at: www.cdc.gov.

CHAPTER 14:
MEDICATION STORAGE AND DISPOSAL

When it comes to keeping medications safe and getting rid of them properly, every detail matters to protect your health and the environment. I'm going to teach you the art and science of storing your medications safely and correctly so that they stay safe and effective. We will talk about the best ways to get rid of all kinds of medications, from expired pills to unused treatments, in a way that is both responsible and good for the environment. To keep you and others safe, I will also show you the best ways to get rid of sharps like needles and lancets. Join me in this chapter as we look at some of the most important but often forgotten parts of managing medications and how they help keep your family and the community healthy. You'll be able to keep track of your medicine's lifecycle with clear instructions, making sure it's safe and effective at all times.

14.1: Proper Storage Techniques

Let's learn a little more about how to store medications properly. I'm here to help you store medications correctly so that you get the most out of them. Here are some pro tips, important things to keep in mind, and real-life examples to help you keep your medications in good condition.

Best Places to Store:
Think outside the (medicine) box. A cool, dry place is best, but consider details like a locked medicine cabinet or a dedicated box in your bedroom's

closet. To keep things stable and avoid confusion, always keep medications in their original package when possible.

The Refrigeration Rule:
Medications like insulin, some eye drops, and liquid antibiotics need to be refrigerated to stay stable and effective. A good rule of thumb is if the medication comes refrigerated from the pharmacy, that's how you should keep it at home. And don't forget that it shouldn't be too cold – the butter compartment is a safe bet for avoiding freezing.

Childproofing:
Safety caps are great, but curious little hands can be surprisingly nimble. For extra safety, consider putting the medication in a locked box or on a high shelf in the closet. It's important to keep these medications out of sight and out of reach.

Knowing About Expiration Dates:
Did you know that EpiPens lose some of their efficacy when they are past their expiration date? This could make them less useful in an emergency. Mark the dates that things go bad so you can see them, and set alarms to tell you to check your stock.

Sunlight and Medications:
Just like sunlight can hurt your skin, it can also break down the active ingredients in medications like tetracycline antibiotics, which means they work less well and may contain dangerous byproducts. Never put medications out in the sun or on a windowsill; always put them in a drawer or closet.

How to Travel Smart with Meds:
Extreme temperature changes in checked bags can damage medications. You should keep medications in your carry-on, preferably in a small, insulated medical bag. For instance, if you need to bring biologics like Enbrel with you on a trip, put it in a sealed bag with a cold pack and let security know you have the medication with you.

SPECIAL CONSIDERATIONS FOR
MEDICATION STORAGE

Liquid medicines:
Although many medications need to be refrigerated, not all do. Double-check the bottle. Original bottles usually state whether the medication needs to be refrigerated. If the medication was not refrigerated at the pharmacy when you picked it up, do not refrigerate it at home.

Ointments and Creams:
These should not be kept in warm, damp places. Otherwise, the ingredients will separate and break down. A cool, dry drawer in the bedroom works best.

Inhalers:
Exposure to extreme temperatures can affect the propellant and medication delivery. Keep them away from direct heat and at room temperature.

14.2: Safe Disposal of Medications

Disposing of medications responsibly is just as important as storing them correctly. Here's how to do it:

Drug Take-Back Programs in Your Area

> **Hack:** Sites like DisposeMy-Meds.org have searchable lists that can help you find places to get rid of your medications.

A drug take-back program is the best way to get rid of medications that are no longer needed or have passed their expiration date. These programs are the safest way to get rid of most medications. Places like community health centers, hospitals, and police offices have drug take-back programs that make it safe to get rid of old or unused medications. Some pharmacies have mail-back programs or other ways to get rid of medications. Talk to your pharmacist to see if they offer any services that can help you get rid of your medicines safely.

DEA-Authorized Collectors
The Drug Enforcement Administration (DEA) keeps a list of authorized collectors whom you can visit to dispose of medications all year long safely. You can find a collection or drop-off spot near you by visiting the DEA's Diversion Control Division website.

Local Pharmacies
Many pharmacy locations are authorized DEA collectors and are equipped with drug disposal bins so customers can dispose of their medications safely. To find a pharmacy with a disposal bin near you, check with local pharmacies or visit their websites for more information. It's important to remove all personal health information (PHI) from medication labels or packaging before disposal. Please note that these bins may have restrictions on the types of medications they can accept, typically not allowing illicit substances and certain high-risk medications like Opioids.

The FDA's "Flush List"
Certain medicines may pose a greater risk to others and have specific instructions to be flushed down the sink or toilet when no longer needed and if a take-back option is not available. Check the medication label or patient information paper, or look at the FDA's list of medications that should be flushed to see if yours should be. Remember, only flush medicines that are on the FDA's flush list. You can find this information on the FDA's official website. It includes certain opioids and other high-risk drugs that need to be thrown away immediately if not in use.

Household Trash Disposal
If the medication isn't on the list of things that can be flushed, you can throw it away in the trash by following these steps:

1. Mix the drugs with something undesirable, like dirt, used coffee grounds, or cat litter.
2. Put this mix in a bag or container that you can close to keep it from spilling, such as a Ziploc bag.
3. Remove any personal information on the drug packaging; make sure to take this information off prior to throwing it away.

National Prescription Drug Take-Back Day

This is an event held twice a year by the DEA that lets people easily and privately dispose of unwanted drugs. Visit TakeBackDay.dea.gov for information on these events and where they easily and privately dispose of unwanted drugs. Visit TakeBackDay.dea.gov for information on these events and where they occur.

SPECIAL DISPOSAL TIPS
FOR SPECIFIC MEDICATIONS

Inhalers:
Due to their pressurized containers, it can be hard to get rid of inhalers and aerosol products. If you puncture or burn them, they could be dangerous, so many can't be thrown in the trash or recycling bin. If you want to get rid of an inhaler or spray product, read the label and follow the steps given. Contact your local waste management or recycling facility for guidelines on proper disposal, or ask your local pharmacy for guidance.

Patches:
Medication patches, like nicotine patches, must be folded into itself, in half with the sticky sides touching each other and preferably returned to a take-back program. If you have to throw them away, make sure they are in a bag and out of reach of pets and kids. Used or extra fentanyl patches should be flushed to prevent accidental exposure due to how strong and dangerous the remaining medications can be.

Biologics:
Injection treatments like Humira and Enbrel usually come with containers to get rid of sharp objects. When they are full, these buckets can be taken back to a program that takes them back or thrown away according to the rules in your area for sharps.

Controlled and Narcotic Medications:
These medications carry a high risk of abuse and accidental poisoning. Whenever possible, they should be returned to a take-back program. If you have to get rid of them at home and they're not on the FDA's flush list,

follow the trash disposal guidelines. But you might want to disable them first by soaking them in water and mixing them with kitty litter to stop anyone from misusing them.

14.3: Sharps Disposal Guidelines

Getting rid of sharps like needles, syringes, and lancets safely is an important part of taking care of your health at home. If you need help getting rid of these possibly dangerous items safely, I'm here to help.

Knowing How Important It Is

If sharps are not discarded properly, they could hurt or endanger people in your home, sanitation workers, and even the environment. Getting rid of sharps the right way lowers these risks and ensures they don't harm anyone or contribute to pollution.

STEPS FOR SAFE DISPOSAL PRACTICES

1. **Secure a Sharps Disposal Container:**
   The first thing you should do is get a sharps disposal container that the FDA has approved. These containers are made to hold these items safely. These cases can't be punctured, and the lids fit tightly to keep sharps inside. You can get these containers online, at pharmacies, or medical supply stores.

   > **Hack:** www.safeneedledisposal.org offers a searchable database of sharps disposal locations by zip code across the United States, including pharmacies, hospitals, clinics, and public facilities.

2. **Filling the Container**
   It's important not to fill up your sharps container all the way. Aim to dispose of it when it's about three-quarters full to prevent accidents.

3. **Correctly Sealing the Container**
   Once the container is full, make sure the lid is tight and reinforced so that any sharps don't get out while it's being thrown away.

4. **Finding Disposal Sites**
   Disposal methods may vary based on your location. You can find disposal sites by searching "sharps disposal" on the FDA.gov website.

COMMON DISPOSAL
SITE OPTIONS

Drop-off Collections:
Certain fire stations, police departments, hospitals, clinics, and even select pharmacies offer sharps disposal services. There are also designated drop-off points at some community centers or local health departments.

Mail-back Services:
Certain programs let you mail your container to a disposal facility equipped to handle sharps. These services usually offer pre-paid packaging that meets safety regulations.

Community Collection Events:
Look for community-wide collection events put on by your local health department or waste management services. At these events, you can bring your filled sharps container for safe disposal.

Throwing sharps in household trash, recycling bins, or down the toilet raises the risk of injury and contaminating the environment. Regular plastic can be punctured, so it's not recommended to use any container that is not designed for sharps disposal.

STEPS FOR ALTERNATIVE SOLUTIONS
FOR SHARPS DISPOSAL

Let's say you can't find a sharps disposal container that the FDA has approved. That being said, you need to find a safe way to deal with your sharps waste until you can get one. Here's what you can do:

1. **Use a Heavy-Duty Plastic Container**
   Find a strong, heavy-duty plastic container with a lid that fits tightly on top. Bottles of cleaning detergent, bleach, or other rigid plastic containers are good examples. Make sure the container is not easily breakable and has a screw-on cap or a lid that snaps firmly in place to keep it from opening by accident.

2. **Label the Container**
   Make sure everyone in your home knows what's in the container by clearly labeling it with a warning like "Sharps – Do Not Recycle." This way, no one will handle or throw away the container by accident.

3. **Safe Storage**
   Keep kids and pets away from the container. Store in a cool, dry place and in an upright position so that it doesn't leak or get punctured.

4. **Do Not Overfill**
   Do not fill the container more than three-quarters of the way to the top so that sharps do not poke through or the lid does not fit firmly. This helps prevent needle-stick injuries when handling the container.

5. **Seal and Tape the Container**
   Once the container reaches the fill line, secure the lid tightly and tap it down with heavy-duty tape to ensure it stays closed by securing it tightly and taping it down with heavy-duty tape.

Remember that these steps are only temporary until you can get a sharps container that the FDA has approved. To make sure that sharps waste is thrown away safely, get the right container as soon as possible.

For additional information and resources regarding finding local disposal options, visit the FDA and Environmental Protection Agency (EPA) websites. Your local public health department's website can also be a valuable resource for locating disposal options and learning about local regulations.

Wrapping it all up...

Properly storing and disposing of your medications ensures they help rather than harm. Take-back programs are the gold standard for disposal. As a backup, the FDA's guidelines for flushing and trash disposal are there to keep everyone safe. Extra care needs to be taken with sharps and controlled substances to safeguard not only our health and safety but also the well-being of our community and the environment.

FURTHER READING FOR CHAPTER 14:
MEDICATION STORAGE AND DISPOSAL

U.S. Food and Drug Administration (FDA)
For guidelines on proper storage techniques and safe disposal of medications, including how to dispose of unused medicines, visit the U.S. Food and Drug Administration.
Available at: www.fda.gov.

Environmental Protection Agency (EPA)
Learn about environmentally safe medication disposal methods to prevent pollution and protect wildlife from the Environmental Protection Agency.
Available at: www.epa.gov.

Safe Needle Disposal
For comprehensive guidelines on the proper disposal of sharps, including syringes and lancets, refer to Safe Needle Disposal's website.
Available at: www.safeneedledisposal.org.

CHAPTER 15:
TRAVELING WITH MEDICATIONS

Take a deep breath and relax as we go over the basics of traveling with medications. This is an important part for anyone who wants to stay healthy while traveling. I'm here to be your guide and show you how to get medications ready for travel so that you always have what you need, no matter where you are in the world. I'll help you get through airport security and make sure your medications are packed and displayed in a way that makes them easy to check as you travel. Although it may be challenging to adjust your medication schedule when you're in a different time zone, we'll talk about ways for you to stay on track with your health routine no matter what time it is where you are. And don't worry if you ever get caught without your medications—I'll give you useful tips on how to handle this situation, too. Step into this chapter, and let's make your travel experience seamless and safe, with your health needs perfectly managed every step of the way.

15.1: Travel Preparation

You need to carefully plan your trip to ensure that you don't have to stop your health routine while traveling with medications. No matter where your adventures take you, here's how to ensure that your trip goes smoothly and your health is taken care of.

Ask for a Vacation Override:
If you need to take longer than the time your prescription is due to be refilled, talk to your pharmacy about a vacation override. This lets you get your prescription refilled early, making sure you have enough medication for the whole trip.

Keep a Medication List:
Keep a detailed list of your medications, including their brand names, how much you should take, and how to reach the doctor who prescribed them. This list is very helpful in case of an emergency or if you need to see a doctor while you're away.

Pack an Extra Supply:
Pack an additional supply of medication in case your trip is delayed or longer than planned. Having extra means you won't have to worry about running out, especially if you're in a place where medication might not be easy to get to.

EXTRA TIPS
FOR TRAVEL PREPARATION

Keep in Original Packaging:
Always bring medications with you in their original, labeled containers to avoid any questions or issues at security checks.

Pack in Carry-On Luggage:
Make sure that your medications are in your carry-on bag so they stay visible with your checked bags.

Check Legal Restrictions:
Before you go on an international trip, make sure that the medications you are taking are allowed in the country you are going to. The International Narcotics Control Board (INCB) website has information about drug limits around the world.

Carry a Letter from a Healthcare Professional:
For controlled substances or injectable medication, bring a letter from your healthcare provider that explains your situation and why you need to take your medications.

Know your Insurance and drugstore Contacts:
Please remember to bring your prescription insurance card and the phone numbers of your pharmacy and healthcare provider.

15.2: Airport Security Tips

Getting through airport security with medications on you doesn't have to be a stressful part of your trip. You can make sure the process goes smoothly and keep your health in check if you know what to do and plan ahead. Here are some tips that will help you handle medications like a pro at airport security.

Understand TSA Rules:
You can bring solid medications like tablets or capsules with you as long as they are screened by the Transportation Security Administration (TSA). You don't have to put medications in the quart-sized bag.

Liquid Medications:
If you have any liquid medication with you, let the TSA officer know at the start of the screening process. Liquid medicines are allowed in acceptable amounts above the standard 3.4 ounces, and they don't have to be in sealed bags. However, they must be declared to security officers at the checkpoint for inspection.

Declare Your Medications:
You must tell the TSA officer about any liquids, gels, or aerosols that you are carrying. Also, mention any patches, creams, or other unusual forms of medication.

Request a Hand Inspection:
If you don't want your medications to go through the X-ray machine, you can ask for a hand inspection. Make sure you ask for this before the screening process starts.

Keep Contacts Handy:
Keep the contact information, such as the phone number of the U.S. embassy or consulate that is closest to you and the number of the U.S. embassy or consulate that is closest to you, in case you need help while you are traveling.

> **Hack:** Documentation is Key. Keep a copy of your prescriptions, a list of your medications from your pharmacy, or a letter from your doctor that proves you need the medication. This is important if you are going to be traveling internationally or if you need to bring controlled substances like opioids or amphetamine salts with you.

If you follow these tips, you'll have no trouble getting through airport security and can be sure that your medications stay with you and are ready to use during your trip. Remember that the best way to have a smooth experience with the TSA is to be ready and communicate clearly with them.

15.3: Time Zone Adjustments

Going from one time zone to another can be tricky, especially if you need to take your medications on time. Don't worry, though. You can take medication without missing a beat, no matter where you are in the world, as long as you plan ahead and make some smart changes. Here is a simple plan to help you stick to your medication schedule even when you're traveling between time zones.

Know what medications you take
First, you should know which medications need to be taken at certain times and which ones can be taken at different times. For example, medications for heart conditions, diabetes, and seizure disorders often need precise timing

to maintain their effectiveness. On the other hand, medications for conditions like high cholesterol may give you more freedom.

Make plans ahead of time
Before you leave, prepare your medication plan for the time zone you'll be traveling to. Write it down on a calendar. In terms of time, going east means "losing" time, and going west means "gaining" time. This might change how and when you need to take your medications.

Get help from a professional
It can be helpful to talk to your pharmacist or other healthcare provider. They can give you specific advice on how to change your drug schedule based on your plans and the types of medications you take. They can suggest temporarily altering your dosing times or frequency to better align with your new time zone.

Small changes over time
For big time zone changes, you should slowly change the way you take your medications a few days before you leave. This will help your body adjust and have less of an effect on it. Adjusting your schedule by an hour every day before your trip can help things go more smoothly.

Make use of technology
Use technology to keep track of when you need to take your medications. If you move to a new time zone, you can set alarms on your phone or use an app to tell you when it's time to take your next dose. There are times when this can save you when you're exploring new places and your normal pattern is off.

Make medications easy to get to
The best thing to do is to put medications in your carry-on bags. What if your flight is delayed or takes an unexpected turn? You might not be able to get to your checked luggage for longer than planned. Having your medications on hand means you won't miss a dose due to travel hiccups.

Traveling across time zones doesn't have to disrupt your medication regimen. If you plan ahead, are flexible, and get help from your healthcare team, you can enjoy your trip without stress, no matter where you are in the world. The key is preparation and adaptation.

15.4: Emergency Medication Strategies

It can be stressful to be away from home and realize you forgot your medication, but don't worry just yet! I'm here to help you get through this unexpected situation. Here are some things you can do if you forget medications while you're traveling.

Contact Your Pharmacy
First, call your usual pharmacy. Most of the time, moving your medication from one pharmacy to another is easy, especially if you use a national chain. This means your medication regimen doesn't have to skip a beat just because you're away from home. Explain your situation. They can often have your prescription ready for pick-up at a nearby branch in no time. Of course, you are not limited to the same chain; you can also transfer to any local or independent pharmacy where you are staying (see Chapter 1.4 for more information).

Get in touch with your Healthcare Provider
If your pharmacy can't help directly, your next call should be to your healthcare provider. They can send a new prescription to a local pharmacy where you're staying. To speed up the process, make sure you have the phone number and address of a nearby pharmacy ready when you call.

Think about walk-in clinics or urgent care centers.

If you can't reach your regular doctor, especially on the weekends or holidays, you might be able to get help at an urgent care or walk-in clinic. There, a healthcare professional can look at your condition and prescribe medication while you are on your trip.

Know what medications you take
Take a list of your medications with you at all times. The list should include the generic names, dosages, and names of the doctors who prescribed them. This will be very helpful in an emergency when you need to explain your situation to a new healthcare provider or pharmacist.

Plan for Non-Transferable Prescriptions
Certain medications, especially controlled substances, may have stricter regulations that make transfers harder. In these situations, it's best to talk to your doctor or pharmacist about your trip plans ahead of time.

Ask for an Emergency Supply
Depending on the rules of the state or country you're in, pharmacies may be able to give you an emergency supply of medication without a prescription. This typically applies to essential maintenance medications such as those used to treat diabetes or high blood pressure. If you bring your empty bottle to the pharmacist, they can sometimes give you a short-term "holdover" supply. This short-term fix will help you keep up with your health until you can get a proper refill. Remember, this approach is typically more successful within the same pharmacy chain and is usually not available for acute medications like antibiotics or painkillers.

The key is prevention
For future travels, consider packing a small travel health kit with a supply of all your medications. Always keep this kit in your carry-on luggage. Adding a reminder about medications to your packing checklist can prevent this situation from happening again.

Remember, Stay Calm
Even though it's stressful to forget medication, remember that there are ways to get help. Healthcare professionals understand that this can happen and are there to help you get the medications that you need.

Realizing you forgot your medication can be stressful, but with these steps, you'll find that resolving the issue is more straightforward than it might initially seem.

Wrapping it all up...

Traveling should be about having fun and making memories, not worrying about your medications. With these tips in mind and some planning ahead, you can take care of your health needs no matter where your trips take you. Remember that your pharmacist is always available to help if you have any concerns or questions about the medications you take before a trip. Safe travels, and here's to health and adventure!

FURTHER READING FOR CHAPTER 15:
TRAVELING WITH MEDICATIONS

Transportation Security Administration (TSA)
For essential tips on navigating airport security with medications, including what to expect and how to prepare, visit the Transportation Security Administration.
Available at: www.tsa.gov.

Centers for Disease Control and Prevention (CDC)
Access comprehensive travel health information, including how to manage medications when crossing time zones, from the Centers for Disease Control and Prevention.
Available at: www.cdc.gov/travel.

International Society of Travel Medicine (ISTM)
For detailed guidelines on travel preparation and handling medications during travel, consult resources available from the International Society of Travel Medicine.
Available at: www.istm.org.

American Society of Health-System Pharmacists (ASHP)
Learn about emergency medication strategies for travelers, including how to plan for unexpected medical needs while away from home, at the American Society of Health-System Pharmacists.
Available at: www.ashp.org.

CHAPTER 16:

VACCINATIONS AND YOUR HEALTH

This chapter is all about vaccinations, the unsung heroes of our healthcare journey. In addition to keeping us safe, they also keep communities safe from many diseases. I'm here to guide you through the seamless vaccination process available right at your local pharmacy. I'll cover the different types of common vaccinations offered, from flu shots to tetanus, as well as share why and how important they are for your health and the health of the public. Additionally, I'll also talk about the important topic of travel vaccines, your ultimate passport to health, ensuring you're well-protected on your global adventures. This chapter will help you understand the power and importance of vaccinations, debunk myths about them, and celebrate them as important parts of our plan for lifelong health and wellness.

16.1: Vaccination Process in Pharmacies

The process of getting a vaccination at the pharmacy is smooth and convenient, designed to protect your health with minimal disruption to your day. Getting vaccinated at the pharmacy is easy, just like the process of dropping off and picking up a prescription. Plus, you get an added boost to your immune system. Here's a closer look at how it works, whether you're walking in or scheduling an appointment ahead of time.

Walk-ins are welcome

Many pharmacies offer walk-in vaccination services, which makes it easier than ever to stay up to date on your shots. Here's what to expect:

1. **Get there and check-in**
   You'll start by checking in at the pharmacy, just like when you drop off a prescription. Most shots don't need a prescription, so this is a quick step. Bring your ID, your insurance card, and any proof that you've been immunized in the past. For an easier process, wear something easy to get your arms vaccinated. Before you go in, don't forget to eat something and drink some water—it can help make your experience more comfortable.

2. **Vaccination Form:**
   You'll be asked to fill out a vaccination form. This form asks important questions about your health to make sure that the vaccine is safe for you. This step is similar to the first meeting step in the medication process, but it is specific to shots.

3. **Verification of insurance**
   The pharmacy team will check to see if your insurance covers the vaccine, which is similar to how they check prescription benefits. It can be hard to understand insurance, but most plans cover a lot of different shots. Not sure what's covered? Call your insurance or check online.

4. **Getting the shot**
   A licensed pharmacist or certified technician will give the shot after all the paperwork and insurance issues are taken care of. This step is like "pick-up" in the prescription process, but instead of leaving with a drug, you get your shot right then and there.

> **Hack:** If you're uninsured or your plan doesn't cover a vaccine, don't worry. Ask us about discount programs or check if there are any government or manufacturer programs available.

5. **Observation after vaccination**

   In accordance with CDC standards, you may be asked to wait for a short time to be watched to ensure you don't have any immediate reactions. This is a normal safety step, like being told about possible side effects when you pick up your prescription. If you do react later on, it's important to report it through the Vaccine Adverse Event Reporting System (VAERS).

   > **Hack:** The Centers for Disease Control and Prevention (CDC) website has resources and links to each state's immunization registry that give detailed guidance on how to get to vaccination records. You can get specific instructions and direct links to your immunization history or the immunization history of a patient on the CDC's Immunization Registries page. This ensures that both patients and healthcare providers have the necessary information to make informed healthcare decisions and maintain comprehensive care.

6. **Appointments to Make Things Easy:**

   If you'd rather plan, many pharmacies also let you make an appointment for your vaccination. This makes sure there are few lines and that the process goes smoothly. It's the same process, but you have to choose an exact time slot that works for you.

7. **Talking and writing things down:**

   Just like when you pick up your medications, your pharmacist will talk to you after giving you the vaccine. You can ask questions and find out about possible side effects and what to expect after getting vaccinated. You'll be given paperwork to keep for your notes after getting your shot, which is especially helpful if you need to travel or go to school.

ACCESSING VACCINATION RECORDS

When you get a vaccine at a pharmacy, the information is recorded and sent to a state immunization register. This ensures that your complete vaccination history is kept up to date. Healthcare providers and patients can access this information through the state's health department's website. This easier access helps keep vaccine records up to date, avoid duplicate vaccinations, and ensure that no shots are missed.

The process of getting vaccinated at the pharmacy combines the ease and familiarity of getting a prescription filled with the important health benefit of staying immunized. Walk-ins are welcome, and they're great for last-minute or on-the-spot vaccination needs. But if you prefer to avoid waiting, booking an appointment can save you time. Many pharmacies now let you schedule appointments online or through handy apps, complete with reminders for your second dose if you're getting a vaccine that requires a follow-up.

16:2: Common Vaccinations

Getting a vaccine at your local pharmacy is an easy and convenient way to protect your health and the health of those around you. Today's pharmacies offer a wide range of vaccines to provide vaccination needs for a wide range of individuals and health conditions. I'm here to help you find your way through the different vaccinations commonly offered at your local pharmacy, making it easier for you to meet your vaccination needs.

Influenza (Flu) **Vaccine:**
This vaccine is very important for preventing flu-related sickness and serious health problems. It is recommended once a year for people ages six months and up.

Tdap (Tetanus, Diphtheria, Pertussis) **Vaccine:**
This is recommended for adults who haven't had this vaccine since they were teens and pregnant mothers in their third trimester. A Td (tetanus and diphtheria) booster shot is recommended every ten years.

Shingles Vaccine (Shingrix):
This vaccine is recommended for adults aged 50 and up to protect them from getting shingles, a painful skin disease characterized by a rash.

Pneumococcal Vaccine:
This vaccine protects against pneumococcal diseases like pneumonia in adults over 65 and people with certain health conditions like diabetes as well as heart and lung diseases.

Hepatitis A and B Vaccines:
These vaccinations are for individuals who are more likely to get these infections, such as travelers and people with chronic liver conditions.

Human Papillomavirus (HPV) Vaccine:
This vaccine protects against diseases related to HPV, including certain cancers. It is recommended for teens and adults up to 26 years old and, in some cases, up to 45 years old.

COVID-19 Vaccine:
This is recommended for individuals aged 12 and up to protect against COVID-19 and its complications. According to the latest health guidelines, booster doses are recommended to maintain immunity.

Respiratory Syncytial Virus (RSV) Vaccine:
This vaccine is suggested for older people and certain high-risk groups to protect against the Respiratory Syncytial Virus (RSV), which is a major cause of respiratory illnesses in older adults and individuals with chronic conditions or underlying health issues

WHO SHOULD GET VACCINATED?

At every stage of life, getting vaccinated is an important way to stay healthy. Here is a quick rundown of who should get vaccinated:

Young children and kids in school:
It's important to follow the pediatric vaccination schedule to protect children against diseases like measles and whooping cough.

Adults 50 Years and Up:
Because of the higher risk associated with aging, older adults should get the shingles vaccine when they are 50 years old or older and the pneumococcal vaccine when they are 65 years old or older.

International travelers:
People planning to travel internationally should get vaccinated prior to travel to protect themselves against diseases like typhoid and hepatitis A, which rundown are more common in destination countries.

People with Long-Term Health Problems:
Individuals with heart disease or other chronic health issues should get flu and pneumococcal shots as soon as possible to avoid complications.

Women who are pregnant:
Pregnant women are recommended to get the Tdap vaccine in order to protect themselves and their newborns from whooping cough.

During Pandemics or Outbreaks:
Staying updated with vaccines like COVID-19 and RSV becomes even more important during pandemics and outbreaks to stop the spread and harm of these viruses.

With flexible hours and, often, no appointment necessary, pharmacies now make it easier to get vaccinated. Unsure about which vaccines are right for you or your family? Contact or visit your local pharmacy to ask questions, get vaccinated, or find out about the newest vaccine recommendations.

16.3: Vaccine Importance

One of the most important things that public health has done is make vaccines available to everyone. This is because vaccines protect people from diseases that cause widespread illness, disability, or death. I've seen firsthand how vaccinations can impact people's health and the health of their communities. Let's talk about why vaccines are important, the risks of not getting them, and the important safeguard called "herd immunity."

How Vaccines Work

Vaccines work by making our immune systems think they are infected with a disease, which makes them build up defenses without actually giving us the disease. By getting ready for the disease, your body will be ready to fight it off if you're ever exposed to the actual disease, which could keep you from getting sick or make it much less severe. This is why everyone should think about getting vaccinated.

Vaccines prevent diseases and protect against measles, polio, tetanus, the flu, and many more, all of which can be very dangerous and life-threatening. Thanks to widespread vaccination efforts, they also save lives, making many diseases that used to be common and deadly rare or eradicated in parts of the world.

WHAT COULD GO WRONG
IF YOU DON'T GET VACCINATED

What happens when you decide not to get vaccinated affects more than just you; it can affect your family and the community as a whole.

Disease Vulnerability:
People who haven't been vaccinated are more likely to get and spread infectious diseases.

Complications and Major Outcomes:
If you don't get vaccinated, diseases can lead to serious health problems, hospitalization, and even death.

The Strain on Healthcare Systems:
Outbreaks of preventable diseases can overload healthcare facilities, taking resources away from other patients who need urgent care.

HERD IMMUNITY:
A COLLECTIVE SHIELD

When the majority becomes immune to a disease, it's not likely to spread from person to person. This is called "herd immunity." This kind of community protection can help shield people who can't get vaccinated, like newborns, people with certain health problems, or people whose immune systems aren't strong enough.

Community Protection:
When you get vaccinated, you're not only protecting yourself but also helping to protect people around you who may be more likely to get sick.

Limits Outbreaks:
High vaccination rates help control and get rid of infectious diseases, stop breakouts before they happen, and protect public health.

Special Considerations:
Herd immunity can help protect people who haven't been vaccinated, but it could be better. Outbreaks do happen, especially in places where people are less likely to have been vaccinated. This risk reminds us how important it is for the majority of people to get vaccinated.

Getting vaccinated is an important part of staying healthy and keeping the public safe. They stop diseases from spreading, lower the cost of health care, and save lives. Even though herd immunity helps protect our communities, it only works when the majority gets vaccinated. As your pharmacist, I want you to stay well-informed, talk to your healthcare providers, and consider the many ways that getting vaccinated can help you and the people around you. We can make the future healthy and safer for everyone if we all work together.

16.4: Travel Vaccines

When planning a trip, especially one that takes you outside of the country, it's important to consider both what to pack and how to stay healthy. I'm here to help you understand the world of travel vaccines so that you are as ready for your trip as you are for your health.

Getting travel vaccines is the best way to protect yourself from diseases that aren't common where you live but are very dangerous where you're going. Getting certain vaccines may be necessary, depending on where you're going. For example, people who want to go to warm areas might need to get shots for hepatitis A and B, yellow fever, or typhoid. People who want to go to parts of Africa or South America might need to get a meningitis vaccine. The key vaccines often considered for travelers include:

Hepatitis A and B:
Hepatitis can cause liver damage, and these shots can protect you from the two most common kinds. Vaccination against Hepatitis A is recommended for travelers to countries where sanitation and hygiene may be poor, and Hepatitis B vaccination is recommended for travelers who might be at increased risk of exposure through medical treatment, sexual contact, or potential exposure to blood products.

Typhoid Fever:
This is especially important if you're going to a place where the water or food safety standards aren't very good.

Yellow Fever:
To enter some countries, such as Africa and South America, you need to show proof that you've had this vaccine.

Japanese Encephalitis and Rabies:
Consider these if you're planning extended travel or activities outside, especially in rural areas.

Meningococcal disease:
Vaccination against meningococcal disease is especially recommended for travelers who plan to travel to regions where the disease is common, such as travelers who are going to Sub-Saharan Africa and some places in the Middle East or for those participating in certain activities that increase their risk.

Who should take them?
Someone traveling to regions where these diseases are prevalent should consider the vaccines. Your healthcare provider, pharmacist, or travel medicine specialist can provide advice based on your medications, your destination, and the activities you plan to do.

When should I get vaccinated?
It's important to plan because some vaccines need to be given weeks or even months before your trip to work. You can stop by the pharmacy or schedule a consultation with your local pharmacist or your healthcare provider well before you leave. They can talk about your travel plans, look over your history of immunizations, and make sure you have all the necessary vaccinations to make your trip as pleasant and risk-free as possible.

There are so many things to do when you travel, and if you plan, you can make sure you enjoy every moment healthily and safely. Getting the right vaccinations can make all the difference, whether you're visiting old ruins, trekking through rainforests, or just relaxing on a beach in the middle of nowhere.

Hack: The Centers for Disease Control and Prevention (CDC) website (www.cdc.gov/travel) is a great place to find out more. It gives you specific information on the vaccines you should get based on where you're going, as well as health warnings and tips for staying healthy while you're away. The World Health Organization (WHO) website (www.who.int) also has information about world health and suggestions for vaccines.

16.5: Free Vaccine Resources

Getting the vaccinations you need might seem difficult for people without health insurance, but there are many ways to get these important services for little or no cost. Knowing where to find these resources and how to use them can help protect your health and prevent the spread of diseases.

Vaccines for Children (VFC) Program

The VFC program is a lifesaver for those under 18 by giving free immunizations to children who are eligible for Medicaid, don't have insurance, or whose insurance doesn't cover them. Clinics and pediatric offices that are part of the VFC program provide vaccines according to the recommended immunization schedule. You can learn more and locate nearby VFC providers by visiting the Centers for Disease Control and Prevention (CDC) dedicated VFC webpage at (www.cdc.gov/vaccines/programs/vfc/index.html).

Health Departments in your town and state

Many local and state health departments have immunization programs that let residents, even those without health insurance, get vaccinations for free or at a low cost. These departments are very important for public health measures to stop disease outbreaks and make it easy for people to get vaccinated against flu, hepatitis, HPV, and other diseases. There will be information about immunization programs on the website of your local or state health service. You can use the National Association of County and City Health Officials (NACCHO) at (www.naccho.org/membership/lhd-directory) to find the health department in your area.

Federally Qualified Health Centers (FQHCs)

FQHCs, also known as community health centers, offer a range of health services with fees that vary based on the patient's ability to pay. This means that if you don't have health insurance or can't afford to pay, you may be able to get your vaccinations for free or at a reduced cost. These centers offer vaccinations among their services, which are important for people who live in areas that don't have enough medical care. You can use the locator tool on the Health Resources and Services Administration (HRSA) website by following (findahealthcenter.hrsa.gov) to find a community health center near you.

Pharmacy Programs
Some pharmacies offer free vaccination programs, especially during public health campaigns. Major pharmacy chains sometimes work with health organizations to give people who don't have health insurance free flu shots and other vaccines, such as those for shingles or pneumonia. You can call, visit, or look at their official websites to find out more about these programs and who is eligible.

Charitable Organizations and Clinics
Non-profits like the American Red Cross and local charitable health clinics for uninsured and low-income people often organize free vaccine clinics. These events are typically advertised in community centers, local newspapers, and online community boards, as well as on their websites or through local media. Checking the websites of these organizations or calling them can provide information on upcoming events.

School-based Health Centers
Children in school can typically get free vaccinations at health centers attached to the schools, especially in areas with low incomes. These centers aim to make it easier for people to get medical care, like vaccinations. They offer a range of vaccines, including those for flu, HPV, and other diseases. You can usually find out about the services that school-based health centers offer on school district websites or by contacting the schools directly.

Community Outreach and Health Fairs
Getting vaccinated is often free at community health fairs and outreach programs. Hospitals, health departments, or community organizations that want to improve public health often put on these events. Health fairs and community vaccine events are often advertised in local community centers, churches, and municipal websites. Keeping an eye on community bulletin boards, both online and in physical locations, can also alert you to upcoming opportunities.

Getting vaccinated regularly is important for everyone's health, but it's especially important for people without insurance. The resources outlined above make it possible to get needed vaccinations for free or at a low cost, so money problems don't prevent people from getting important preventive health care.

Wrapping it all up...

A big part of keeping yourself and your community healthy is getting vaccinated. Your neighborhood pharmacy can make it as easy as possible for you to do so. So, next time you're picking up a prescription or just passing by, remember that your local pharmacy is also your go-to spot for vaccinations. If you need to make an appointment or have questions about travel vaccines, they've got some answers and can provide the support you need. Stay healthy and safe travels!

FURTHER READING FOR CHAPTER 16:
VACCINATIONS AND YOUR HEALTH

Centers for Disease Control and Prevention (CDC)
For detailed information on common vaccinations, their importance, and guidelines for both routine and travel vaccines, visit the Centers for Disease Control and Prevention.
Available at: www.cdc.gov/vaccines.

World Health Organization (WHO)
Explore global perspectives on vaccine safety, effectiveness, and public health policies from the World Health Organization.
Available at: www.who.int/health-topics/vaccination.

American Pharmacists Association (APhA)
Learn about the process of vaccination in pharmacies, including how pharmacists are trained and authorized to administer vaccines.
Available at: www.pharmacist.com/immunization.

Travel.State.Gov – U.S. Department of State
For information on required and recommended travel vaccines based on your destination, consult the U.S. Department of State's travel pages.
Available at: www.travel.state.gov/content/travel/en/international-travel/before-you-go/your-health-abroad.html.

Vaccines.gov
Discover resources on where to find free vaccinations and how to access them through federal and state programs in the United States.
Available at: www.vaccines.gov.

CHAPTER 17:
LAB TEST AND MEDICATION IMPACT

In this chapter, you'll learn about the interesting world of lab tests and how they interact with medications. I'm here to clear up the mysteries of common lab tests by telling you what they measure and how they reflect your health. I'll help you understand the complicated language of lab results and turn the numbers and terms that are hard to understand into information that is clear and useful. We'll also talk about the complicated ways that medications can affect these tests and ways to deal with them so that your lab tests accurately reflect your health status, so you can learn more about health care and take a more active role in your health journey.

17.1: Common Lab Tests

Learning about lab tests can be like learning a new language, but it's an important part of taking care of your health. I'm here to break down what these tests measure in a way that is simple to understand. Here are some common lab tests that your doctor might order, why they're done, and what they're looking for.

Complete Blood Count (CBC)
This test measures the red blood cells (RBCs), white blood cells (WBCs), hemoglobin, hematocrit, and platelets in your blood. It is a basic test that can detect signs of illnesses like anemia, infections, and even more serious issues like leukemia.

Lipid Panel
Do you remember hearing your doctor say that they'll check your cholesterol levels? That's what a lipid panel does. It checks how much triglycerides, total cholesterol, "bad" cholesterol (LDL), "good" cholesterol (HDL), and "bad" cholesterol (LDL) are in your blood. This test is key in telling how likely you are to get heart disease.

Basic Metabolic Panel (BMP)
The BMP is a quick look at your body's chemical balance and metabolism. Blood urea nitrogen (BUN) and creatinine are kidney function markers that are checked. Ions such as sodium (Na), potassium (K), chloride, and bicarbonate are also checked. This test helps monitor diabetes, heart disease, and high blood pressure.

Thyroid Function Tests
These tests, which include TSH (Thyroid Stimulating Hormone), T3, and T4, check your thyroid gland's health. They can help determine whether someone has hypothyroidism (an underactive thyroid) or hyperthyroidism (an overactive thyroid).

Liver Function Tests (LFTs)
LFTs measure different enzymes, proteins, and chemicals in your blood to determine your liver's health. They can detect liver disease or damage by testing enzymes like ALT and AST, bilirubin, and albumin. This test is very important for people who have had liver disease in the past or who take medications that affect the liver.

Hemoglobin A1c
This test shows blood sugar levels averaged over the last two to three months, which is important for identifying and managing diabetes. It also keeps track of how well your diabetes treatment plan is working.

Urinalysis
This test examines the concentration, color, and contents of your urine, such as proteins, glucose, and red and white blood cells, to see if there are any signs of kidney disease, diabetes, urinary tract infections, and more.

Each of these tests contributes to giving a full picture of your health. If you're due for any of these tests or if your doctor has recommended them, knowing why they are done can help you feel more in control of your health care.

17.2: Interpreting Lab Results

Let's talk about those lab tests you may have gathered from seeing your doctor. All of those numbers and medical terms can be hard to understand. But don't worry—I'll help you make sense of them, focusing on some common tests. Though these ranges can vary slightly based on the lab, I'll give you a general idea of what's normal and what's not. Always talk with your healthcare provider about your results for personalized advice.

COMPLETE BLOOD COUNT (CBC):

Normal Ranges
- White Blood Cells (WBC): 4,500 to 11,000 cells per microliter
- Hemoglobin (Hgb): Men: 13.8 to 17.2 grams per deciliter,

Women: 12.1 to 15.1 grams per deciliter
- Platelets: 150,000 to 450,000 platelets per microliter

Interpretation: High WBC can mean you have an infection, while low hemoglobin can mean you have anemia, and an abnormal platelet count could mean you have a problem with clotting or a blood disease.

LIPID PANEL:

Normal Ranges
- LDL Cholesterol: Less than 100 mg/dL
- HDL Cholesterol: 40 mg/dL or higher
- Triglycerides: Less than 150 mg/dL

Interpretation: High triglycerides, high LDL ("bad" cholesterol), and low HDL ("good" cholesterol) can all make you more likely to develop heart disease.

BASIC METABOLIC PANEL (BMP):

Normal Ranges
- Creatinine: 0.6 to 1.2 mg/dL
- Blood Urea Nitrogen (BUN): 7 to 20 mg/dL

Interpretation: Abnormal levels can mean that your kidneys aren't working right or that your body's fluid and electrolyte balance is off.

THYROID FUNCTION TESTS:

Normal Ranges
- TSH (Thyroid-Stimulating Hormone): 0.4 to 4.0 mIU/L

Interpretation: High TSH indicates hypothyroidism, which means the thyroid is not working properly (underactive thyroid). Low TSH indica-tes hyperthyroidism, which means it is working too much(overactive thyroid).

LIVER FUNCTION TESTS:

Normal Ranges
- AST and ALT usually fall within 7 to 56 units per liter.

Interpretation: High levels can mean that the liver is sick or damaged.

HEMOGLOBIN A1C:

Normal Ranges
- Less than 5.7%

Interpretation: A1c levels between 5.7% and 6.4% can mean you have prediabetes, and levels of 6.5% or higher mean you have diabetes.

URINALYSIS:

Normal
- Clear, yellow urine with no significant protein or glucose.

Interpretation: Possible causes of abnormal readings include a urinary tract infection, kidney disease, or diabetes.

HACKS FOR UNDERSTANDING YOUR LAB TESTS

Keep a Personal Record:
Tracking changes over time can help you and your doctor know more about your health.

Know Your Baseline:
What's normal for most people might not be your "normal." Talk to your healthcare provider about your baseline amounts so that they can compare them.

Keep in mind that these lab tests are just tools that, along with other information, help your doctor make decisions about your health. Don't worry if something's off. It's a starting point for further investigation or for making changes to your care plan. Always reach out to your doctor or pharmacist with questions or concerns about your results.

17.3: Medication Effects on Lab Results

As we explore the complicated relationship between lab tests and medications, it's important to remember that various medications can affect the results of these tests. To help you understand this relationship better, let's examine some common lab tests and medications that may affect their results.

Complete Blood Count (CBC)

Neutropenia is when the number of white blood cells in your blood drops. This can happen with certain medications, such as cancer drugs like cyclophosphamide. This drop in white blood cells makes it more likely to get an infection. Corticosteroids, such as prednisone, may raise the number of white blood cells, which is why they are used when someone is sick to help them feel better faster.

Liver Function Tests (LFTs)

Taking high amounts of medication that affect the liver, such as acetaminophen (Tylenol) and statins (like simvastatin used for high cholesterol), can cause liver damage. Acetaminophen in large amounts can cause the liver enzymes (AST and ALT) to increase. Seeing high liver enzymes is a sign of liver damage.

Kidney Function Tests (KFTs)

High creatinine levels show that the kidneys are not working properly. NSAIDs like ibuprofen can raise creatinine levels, and ACE inhibitors like lisinopril (used for high blood pressure) can affect potassium and creatinine levels.

Blood Glucose Levels

Having higher blood sugar can make it harder to control diabetes. Taking steroids like prednisone and certain drugs used to treat mental illness, like Olanzapine (Zyprexa), can make blood sugar levels go up. This can happen for people with or without diabetes.

Lipid Panel

Triglyceride and cholesterol levels can increase if you take certain diuretics, such as hydrochlorothiazide, and beta-blockers, such as propranolol, which are both used to treat blood pressure. Ritonavir, a medication used to treat HIV, can also raise cholesterol and triglycerides.

Electrolyte Levels
Diuretics like furosemide and ACE Inhibitors like lisinopril can cause electrolyte imbalances. Furosemide causes low sodium or low potassium levels, known as hypokalemia, while lisinopril can increase potassium levels, also known as hyperkalemia.

Thyroid Function Tests
Lithium, a drug used to treat bipolar disorder, and Interferons used for Hepatitis C and some cancers can both affect the way the thyroid works. Lithium can change the levels of the thyroid-stimulating hormone (TSH), which can often lead to hypothyroidism (low thyroid levels). In contrast, Interferons can lead to both hypo- and hyperthyroidism (high thyroid levels).

17.4: Medication and Lab Test Management

Figuring out how medication affects lab tests can be tough, but if you know what to do, you can get the most accurate results. Here are some tips and tricks for handling this well, along with some examples:

Strategic Timing for Test Accuracy:
For certain medications, timing lab tests carefully is important to prevent skewed results. If you're taking statins, like atorvastatin, to treat high cholesterol, your doctor may suggest a fasting blood test first thing in the morning before you take your medication. This helps you get a good reading on your cholesterol levels without your medication influencing your results.

Comprehensive Medication Review:
Before any lab tests, talk to your healthcare provider in detail about all the medications you're taking. This includes over-the-counter antacids that contain magnesium, which might affect your electrolyte balance; aspirin, which can affect clotting factors; and so on. Communicating your medication list ensures that any possible impacts on lab results are taken into account.

The Importance of Hydration:
Staying hydrated is important for lab tests like those that check kidney health. If you don't drink enough water before tests, you might get skewed results because you're dehydrated. If you are taking medications like furosemide and other diuretics, talk to your doctor first about how you can best prepare for your tests since these medications can affect hydration and electrolyte levels.

Keeping a Medication Log:
Write down any changes you've made to your medications recently, especially if you've started new ones, like beta-blockers for high blood pressure. These medications can affect heart rate and other signs of heart health. Keeping track of these changes helps connect them with any lab test results that were not expected.

Educate Yourself on Medication Interactions:
Some medications can significantly affect lab tests. Biotin supplements, for instance, can interfere with hormone tests, which could lead to misleading results. If you are aware of these interactions, you can talk to your doctor and potentially pause taking them before testing.

Active Communication:
Talk to your doctor if you have concerns or questions about your medications and how they might affect upcoming lab tests. For example, if you have diabetes and take metformin, it's important to know how it might impact your blood sugar levels during fasting tests.

Incorporating these practices into your approach to lab tests can help make sure that the results are an accurate reflection of your health, leading to better and more personalized care.

Wrapping it all up…

Now that you know more about them, lab tests won't just be numbers to you. Instead, they will be useful tools that, along with your medications, play a key role in our path to wellness. Remember, these tests are part of your healthcare journey, helping to make sure that your treatments are safe and effective.

FURTHER READING FOR CHAPTER 17:
LAB TESTS AND MEDICATION IMPACT

Lab Tests Online
For comprehensive information on common lab tests, how to interpret lab results, and understanding how medications may affect these tests, visit Lab Tests Online.
Available at: www.labtestsonline.org.

Mayo Clinic
Explore detailed insights on the effects of medications on lab tests and guidelines for managing medications when preparing for lab testing at the Mayo Clinic.
Available at: www.mayoclinic.org.

American Association for Clinical Chemistry (AACC)
For a deeper understanding of lab test processes and how to interpret results, including the impact of medications, consult resources provided by the AACC.
Available at: www.aacc.org.

National Institutes of Health (NIH)
Gain access to scientific studies and articles about the interaction between medications and laboratory tests, and how to manage these factors in clinical settings from the NIH.
Available at: www.nih.gov.

CHAPTER 18:
PHARMACY FAQS AND TROUBLESHOOTING

Step right up to the pharmacy counter, where your questions find answers, and your confusion becomes clearer! In this chapter, I'll help you find your way through the confusing rules of the pharmacy, covering everything from returns to transfers and more. We'll answer the most common questions pharmacists like myself get while working behind the counter, as well as troubleshoot real-world pharmacy problems, offering practical solutions that you can use. This chapter gives you a look at how pharmacies work from behind the scenes. It's meant to give you knowledge and confidence, which in turn will make your time at the pharmacy better and more enjoyable.

18.1: Pharmacy Policies and Procedures

Have you ever felt like you needed a guidebook to help you understand how pharmacies work? Well, consider this chapter to be just that. I'm here to break down some of the most common pharmacy policies—from returns to a few other details you might encounter. Let's take the mystery out of these processes together so that you can feel confident and well-informed when you go to the pharmacy.

UNDERSTANDING RETURNS

Can I return the medication if I no longer need it?
Unfortunately, once a medication leaves the pharmacy, it can't be returned. This is for safety and regulatory reasons, making sure that all medications you and others receive are safe and haven't been tampered with.

> **PRO Tip:** Before you leave the pharmacy, double-check the name, strength, directions, and quantity to make sure you have the correct medication and that you're clear on how to use it. If you have unused medication, ask about local take-back programs or drop-off areas for safe disposal. If you haven't left the pharmacy yet and realize you no longer want or need the medication you just purchased, ask the pharmacist and let them know your situation. They can sometimes help you find a solution and maybe even take the return.

NAVIGATING TRANSFERS

How do I transfer my prescription to another pharmacy?

Transferring a prescription is generally straightforward. Provide the new pharmacy with your current pharmacy's contact information and the details of the prescription you wish to transfer, and they'll handle the rest. (See Chapter 1.5 for more details)

> **PRO Tip:** Controlled substances have stricter transfer rules. The prescription must at least be dispensed once at the original store, then can only be transferred once after. If the prescription has remaining refills, the refills must remain at the new pharmacy and cannot be transferred anywhere else. If you're transferring a controlled medication, it's best to start the process a few days in advance to avoid any interruptions in your medication regimen. If you are going out of town or out of the country, consider asking for a vacation override. For controlled substances, you will need your doctor to approve an early fill and to communicate this approval to the pharmacy.

REFILL POLICIES

What if I need an early refill?

As long as you have remaining refills, an early fill is possible, especially if you plan on paying out-of-pocket (without your insurance) or with a discount card instead. Getting an early refill paid for by insurance will depend on your medication (controlled versus non-controlled) and insurance policy rules. For travel or other special circumstances, pharmacies can request an "override" from your insurance. (See Chapter 1.4 for more details).

> **PRO Tip:** Plan for vacations or changes in your schedule that might affect your medication needs. Contact the pharmacy as soon as you know you'll need an early refill.

CONTROLLED MEDICATIONS

Why are there so many rules for controlled medications?

Because they can be abused, controlled medications are regulated more strictly. Limits on amounts, refill times, and how medications can be received are all part of this.

> **PRO Tip:** Always talk to your pharmacist about your needs for controlled medication and be aware of the rules around them. Your pharmacist can often help guide you on your next steps but know that most actions involving controlled substances, especially those involving early fills, will need your doctor to communicate with the pharmacy team.

INSURANCE ISSUES

What do I do if my insurance won't cover my medication?

Talk to your pharmacy team if you encounter problems with your insurance. They can check to see if you need prior authorization, suggest alternatives, or even help you find programs that will help with the medication cost. (See Chapter 4 and Chapter 5 for more details.)

> **PRO Tip:** Keep your pharmacy informed of any changes, such as insurance, name, address, and contact information. This can help avoid surprises at the counter. Some insurance plans confirm identity using this information; if they're not accurate, the pharmacy can't troubleshoot with the insurance plan to help you.

PHARMACY HOURS AND EMERGENCY NEEDS

What if I need my medication outside of regular pharmacy hours?

In these situations, it's a good idea to know where the 24-hour pharmacies are in your area. If they belong to a pharmacy chain, they can often transfer the medication from the closed pharmacy into their 24-hour store. There might be issues with insurance coverage, but you'll have access to the medication you need, and you can work with the pharmacy to reprocess it through insurance at a later time.

> **PRO Tip:** There are billing windows when it comes to insurance reprocessing, which is often 14 days or less after the medication is dispensed (details vary between insurance plans). If you need to do a rebill for your insurance to pay, do it as soon as possible, and don't wait. Communicate with your pharmacy team about your needs and what you plan to do.

SPECIAL ORDERS

Can my pharmacy order specialty medications for me?

Yes, most pharmacies can order medications that they don't normally have in stock, including certain vaccines or specialty drugs. If ordered before the pharmacy's order cut-off time (typically before 5 p.m.), ordered medications often arrive the next business day (usually in the afternoon). For example, medications ordered on Friday, Saturday, and Sunday will arrive on Monday, whereas a medication ordered on Monday will arrive the next day on Tuesday. (See Chapter 1.6 and Chapter 1.7 for more details.)

> **PRO Tip:** Certain medications might take longer to special order, depending on factors like availability and the type of medication. Some medications may even need to be fulfilled by a separate Specialty Pharmacy. Communicate with your pharmacy team ahead of time. They can help guide you and keep you informed along the way.

PHARMACY LOYALTY PROGRAMS

Should I sign up for my pharmacy's loyalty program?

Signing up for loyalty programs can help you save money and receive other benefits. Although most programs don't directly offset the cost of medication, these perks can offset other costs, such as items you need to purchase over the counter or the cost of delivery. Just make sure you read the terms and conditions.

> **PRO Tip:** To get the most out of your pharmacy needs, take advantage of the loyalty program. Ask a store representative to review the loyalty program with you and provide examples of how you can best benefit from it. Usually, these perks can add up, especially for frequent purchases.

Remember, your pharmacy team is here to help you find your way through the confusing world of healthcare rules and regulations. Don't be afraid to reach out if you have any questions or concerns, whether it's about returning medications, transferring prescriptions, or dealing with problems with your insurance. Your pharmacy team is dedicated to making sure you can get the medications and care you need, with clarity and convenience, every step of the way.

18.2: Answering Common Questions

Here is a list of the most common questions I get, along with their answers and helpful hints to make your time at the pharmacy go smoothly, as well as to shed some light on the mysteries of pharmacy terms and processes.

What is the difference between "refill" and "renewal"?
You can get extra amounts of the medication your doctor gave you without getting a new prescription. This is called a refill. When you run out of refills, you need to renew. This means calling your doctor to get a new prescription because the old one has run out or all of its refills have been used up. (See Chapter 1.4 for more details).

> **PRO Tip:** Keep track of your refills and call your doctor a few weeks before your next one to avoid any gaps in your treatment. Setting your medication on auto-refill will also help. Your pharmacy team will automatically reach out to your doctor to renew your medication once all the refills are used up if the medication is set up for automatic refills.

Why do I need prior authorization for some medications?
Prior authorizations mean that your medication is not currently covered by insurance, but they can be covered if certain requirements are met. This is usually for newer, more expensive medications or for medications where there is a cheaper alternative. In this case, your pharmacy team can inform your doctor that a prior authorization is needed for the prescription that they sent. Your doctor's office then would need to look into what requirements need to be met, which could include additional paperwork, in order for your insurance company to cover the cost. Your insurance plan will then review what was submitted by your doctor's office or pharmacy and decide whether your medication will be covered or not. Once a decision has been made, your insurance will either communicate with you, your doctor, or your pharmacy. (See Chapter 4.2 for more details)

> **PRO Tip:** If your doctor prescribes a medication that needs prior authorization, contact your doctor directly. They might still be review-

ing their faxes, and your reaching out directly can help speed up the process. If you are open to alternative medications, inform your doctor. They might have another medication in mind that doesn't require prior authorization and fits your needs. You can also ask your pharmacist for potential alternatives that are covered by your plan.

Can I get my prescription filled early?

Yes, but getting a medication filled early depends on the type of medication and the rules of your insurance plan. There are tighter rules for controlled substances. Your pharmacist can utilize overrides based on your early refill needs. (See Chapter 1.4 for more details).

> **PRO Tip:** Are you planning a trip? A vacation override is something that most insurance plans let you do. To set it up, call your insurance plan and inform them of your trip, including how long you will be away, then reach out to your pharmacy so that they can prepare your extra refill before your trip.

What's the difference between brand-name and generic drugs?

Generic drugs generally cost less than brand-name medications, and they contain the same active ingredients. Name and looks are often the only things that make them different. (see chapter 5.1 for more details).

> **PRO Tip:** Always check to see if there is a generic form. In the long run, it will save you a lot of money. If your medication is only available as a brand name, ask your pharmacist if there is a manufacturer coupon that you could use.

How do I transfer my prescription to another pharmacy?

To transfer a prescription, call the pharmacy where you'd like to move it to and provide them with the contact information of the pharmacy that currently has your medication. They'll handle the rest. (see chapter 1.5 for more details).

> **PRO Tip:** If you're moving to or from a different state, make sure you talk to the new pharmacy first, especially if you are taking con-

trolled substances. Some states have specific rules about transferring prescriptions.

What should I do if I miss a dose of my medication?
If you miss your dose and need to know how to proceed, call or visit your local pharmacist. They can provide you with advice tailored to you and your medications. For most medications, especially for chronic conditions, don't wait until it's almost time for your next dose to take the missed dose. Instead, take it as soon as you remember (See Chapter 3.3 for more details).

> **PRO Tip:** Set alarms or use an app for your medications to help you remember when to take them. Consistency is key.

How do I dispose of unused medications?
Taking medications to a take-back program is the best way to dispose of them safely. Certain medications can be flushed or disposed of through regular trash, but check the FDA guidelines first (See Chapter 14 for more details).

> **PRO Tip:** Don't keep unused medications lying around; drop them off to prevent misuse. Fire stations, police stations, and select pharmacy locations have designated areas to drop off unused or expired medications.

Why does my medication look different this time?
If the pharmacy switches to a different generic manufacturer, medications may look different. This difference in appearance does not affect how well the medication works. Think of it as the same cookies and cream ice cream but from a different store. (See Chapter 13.2 for more details).

> **PRO Tip:** If you notice any changes in the way your medication looks, talk to your pharmacist first. They can verify that it's the correct one. Your medication bottle will also have a description of how your medication should look. If the name of the medication on the bottle is correct and the description of color, shape, and markings matches what is stated on the bottle, you most likely have the correct medication.

What do I do if I have side effects from my medication?

Tell your doctor or pharmacist about any side effects you are experiencing. Sometimes, the dose may need to be changed, another drug with fewer side effects may be used instead, or a simple lifestyle adjustment can be the fix. (See Chapter 2.3 for more details.)

> **PRO Tip:** Write down your side effects and any details, such as when they happen. Recording what you experience can be very helpful for your healthcare team and can help determine the cause as well as the solution.

How can I save money on my prescriptions?

Talk to your doctor and pharmacist if the cost of your medication is a concern. There might be an alternative, cheaper medication you can take. If you have insurance, getting your medication at a "preferred pharmacy" will get you the lowest co-pay. If you don't have insurance, ask your pharmacy team about discount programs and coupons. Pharmacy shopping can also help you find the cheapest price for your medication if you don't have insurance or if insurance is not covering your medication. (See Chapters 4, 5, and 6 for more details and options on saving money.)

> **PRO Tip:** If you have a high-deductible insurance plan, sometimes it's cheaper to pay for the medication out-of-pocket using a discount program than to go through insurance. Just know that the amount you paid will not go toward your deductible.

Why does my insurance sometimes not cover a medication?

Medication coverage can change due to formulary adjustments or policy updates, which are based on considerations like the medication being non-essential or there's a cheaper alternative. If you are taking essential medications, always review your insurance plan's formulary before renewing. Just because a medication was covered for several years prior doesn't mean it will continue to be covered moving forward. Choose your plan based on the medications they cover. (See Chapter 4 for more details).

> **PRO Tip:** If your insurance doesn't pay for your medication, talk to your doctor or pharmacist about other options, such as alternative medications, or ask your doctor to help you file an appeal with your insurance.

What is a compounding pharmacy?
A compounding pharmacy customizes medications to fit the needs of each patient. For example, they might change the form of the medication from a pill to a liquid or combine multiple medications into one to make it easier for the patient. (See chapter 1.2 for more details)

> **PRO Tip:** A compounding pharmacy may be the best choice if you have unique medication needs, such as allergies to certain dyes or chemicals.

Can I still get my medication if there's a shortage or a backorder?
There are times when there aren't enough medications produced, which results in a shortage or backorder. It means that the medication is temporarily out of stock from suppliers. It can be due to manufacturing issues or increased demand. In this case, talk to your pharmacy team about your options. They can reach out to your doctor and ask for an alternative medication, transfer your prescription to another pharmacy that has it in stock, or place it in perpetual order until it becomes available again. (See Chapter 1.6 and Chapter 1.7 for more details)

> **PRO Tip:** Communication is key. Stay in touch with your pharmacy and doctor's office to navigate shortages proactively. Ask your pharmacist for an estimated wait time and consider alternative medications with your doctor if necessary.

How does a pharmacy handle recalled medications?
Pharmacies keep track of the patients who were given recalled drugs and will contact you with directions if you are one of those people. (See Chapter 13.5 for more details)

PRO Tip: Make sure your pharmacy has up-to-date contact information for you so that they are able to reach you if your medication becomes part of a recall.

What are specialty medications?

These medications are used to treat chronic or complex health conditions, and they often need monitoring, as well as special care when they are handled or given. These medications are usually dispensed through a specialty pharmacy, which would have a dedicated team and specialized pharmacist handling your medication. Typically, you would have an option to get the medication delivered directly to you, or you can pick it up at your local pharmacy. For more details, reach out to your pharmacy team and insurance plan to learn more about the special handling of these medications.

PRO Tip: If you're prescribed a specialty medication, ensure you understand the support and monitoring needed. Your pharmacy may offer services that can help.

If I can't leave my house, how can I get my medications?

Most pharmacies offer delivery services, which is helpful for people who can't leave their homes or have trouble moving around. Local pharmacies may offer same-day options, as well as more affordable 1-2-day options. Reach out to your local pharmacy to ask about delivery options that are available to you. (See Chapter 2.2 for more details)

PRO Tip: Certain pharmacies may offer free delivery through their loyalty program. It may be worth signing up, especially if you are homebound. Just make sure to check the program rules and details.

What should I do if I have an allergic reaction to a medication?

If you think you might be having an allergic reaction (for example, breathing problems, a rash, or swelling), you should get medical help right away. To be prepared, allergy medication, including EpiPens, should be readily available, especially if you have any known allergies.

> **PRO Tip:** If you are allergic to any medications, let your healthcare team, including doctors and pharmacists, know. Always check to make sure that your allergies are in the pharmacy system, and check for potential allergens in new prescriptions.

How can I reduce the number of times I visit the pharmacy to pick up my medications?

Pharmacies can often sync your medications and help you limit the number of visits to the pharmacy. This is called medication synchronization or med sync. The process involves aligning the due dates of your medications, saving you time. Not all medications qualify for the program, and it may not be possible to have only one visit per month. Sometimes, alignment fills (a shorter duration or smaller amount) may be dispensed to help align a medication to other medications that are coming up to be filled.

> **PRO Tip:** Ask your pharmacy about enrolling in a med sync program, especially if you're taking multiple medications and make frequent trips to the pharmacy. Alignment fills might be needed to sync your medications better.

What is a medication therapy management (MTM) session?

As the name suggests, MTM is a service that helps people manage their medications. It involves one-on-one meetings with a pharmacist, during which the patient reviews all of their medications and supplements, and the pharmacist reviews their treatment plan to check for duplications, drug interactions, and potential for improvement. If you're taking a lot of medications or are worried about your regimen, an MTM session might be just what you need.

> **PRO Tip:** MTM is often covered by insurance. Contact your plan or review your benefits package for more details to check if MTM services are available to you. If they are, take advantage of the one-on-one time you have with a pharmacist by scheduling the session and preparing for it.

What can I do to remember to take my medications?
It can be hard to remember to take your dose. Use a pill organizer for the week, set your phone's alarms, or get an app that will remind you to take your medicine. For your medicine to work best, you need to take it at the same time every day. (See Chapter 2.2 and Chapter 3.3 for more details)

> **PRO Tip:** Taking your medication regularly and timely is important for your medication to be most effective. If you miss a dose, reach out to your pharmacist on how to proceed.

What does "take with food" really mean?
Certain medications can hurt the walls of your stomach or work better when taken with food. For medications that indicate this, it's important to eat first so that there is something in your stomach and take your medication preferably immediately after eating.

> **PRO Tip:** If your doctor or pharmacist doesn't say to eat a full meal, a small meal or even a snack like crackers will do.

Can I drink alcohol while taking my medication?
Often, the answer is no. Most medications can't work as well or cause more bad effects or worsen side effects when taken with alcohol. (See Chapter 2.3 and Chapter 3.5 for more details)

> **PRO Tip:** A good rule of thumb is if a medication makes you drowsy, dizzy, or tired, it should not be taken with alcohol. However, other medications interact with alcohol that don't follow this, so always talk to your pharmacist or doctor before combining alcohol with any medications.

Why does the pharmacy ask for my insurance every time?
The pharmacy often keeps a record of your insurance information, so if they ask for it, details about your insurance may have changed. (See Chapter 4 for more information regarding insurance plans.)

> **PRO Tip:** Your name must match what is stated on your insurance card. Remember to update your details when you have a name change, such as after you get married. Keeping your contact information, such as your name, address, and phone number, up to date can help your pharmacy team troubleshoot and even find your insurance coverage.

What if I can't swallow pills?
Difficulty swallowing pills is a common issue. Some tablets can be cut in half or crushed, while capsules can be opened and sprinkled into food like applesauce or yogurt. There are also techniques that you can use to make it easier to swallow as well. (See Chapter 3.4 for more details)

> **PRO Tip:** Always ask your pharmacist before crushing or splitting pills since certain kinds, such as those that are Extended Release (ER) or Controlled Release (CR), often can't be cut or split opened due to safety risks.

Is it safe to use multiple pharmacies?
Using more than one pharmacy can make your care less effective and increase the risk of drug interactions. Each of your medications is checked for drug interactions and duplication by your pharmacist prior to your pick-up for safety. Not having all your medications in one place means your pharmacist can't do a comprehensive check. (See Chapter 1.1 and Chapter 2.4 for more details)

> **PRO Tip:** If possible, stick to one pharmacy. If you must use more than one, make sure that each pharmacy has a complete list of your medications. Remember to share any over-the-counter medications and natural or herbal remedies you might take.

What's the deal with medication expiration dates?
Medications can lose their effectiveness after their expiration date and may even become harmful. It is not recommended to take medications past their expiration date. (See Chapter 3.6 for more details)

> **PRO Tip:** Don't take expired medications. If you have expired meds, bring them to a take-back program or an authorized collector, such as your local fire station or pharmacy, for safe disposal.

What should I do about side effects that get in the way of my daily life?

Side effects can be challenging but manageable. Tell your doctor or pharmacist about them. There might be ways to adjust your medication or its timing to lessen its effects without affecting your treatment. (See Chapter 2.3 and Chapter 3.5 for more details)

> **PRO Tip:** Keep a list or diary of your side effects, including when you experience them, and share these with your doctor or pharmacist. This information is helpful in finding solutions.

Can I still get vaccinated at the pharmacy if I don't have insurance?

Yes, there are many resources available to people who have no insurance or have low income to get vaccinated. (See Chapter 16.5 for more details)

> **PRO Tip:** Pharmacies are the most convenient and available option due to the ability to walk in or make appointments. If you need a vaccine but don't have insurance or your insurance doesn't cover it, ask the pharmacy team for help. They may have a discount program they can apply to help lower your cost.

What should I do if my medication is being returned to stock (RTS) before I am able to pick it up?

If your medication is already ready for pick-up but is at risk of being returned to stock (RTS), contact the pharmacy immediately to let them know you still need it. Pharmacies typically keep a medication available on their shelves for a set period, often 7 to 14 days, after which they return the medication to stock if it's not picked up. Tell them what's going on and ask if they can hold it for a little longer or if they can refill it the next time you can come.

> **PRO Tip:** Having your medication Returned To Stock RTS'd) does not mean your prescription is canceled. It just means the medication itself, not your prescriptions, has returned to stock. You can always call your pharmacy to fill your prescription again if this happens. To prevent this, find out from the pharmacy how long they keep medications and try to pick up your prescriptions within that time frame. Many pharmacies offer services like text or email notifications to remind you when your prescription is ready for pickup. You might also want to set personal reminders to pick up medications or look into home delivery choices if you often have problems getting them on time.

I was told my prescription expired; how long are my prescriptions good for?

How long a prescription is good depends on the type of medication and the state laws. Most non-controlled prescriptions are good for one year from the date they were written. But there are tighter rules for prescriptions for controlled substances: Most Schedule II drugs are only good for 30 days. Schedule III and IV drugs, on the other hand, can be used for up to 6 months. It's important to check the specific expiration dates for your prescriptions and understand the regulations in your state. (See Chapter 1.5 for more details).

> **PRO Tip:** Your medication bottle often includes the expiration date of your prescription, typically shown as "refills valid until [date of expiration]. If not, write down the date the prescription was issued on the label and keep track of when you need to ask for renewal so you don't end up with expired prescriptions. Making an appointment with your doctor on a regular basis can help ensure that your prescriptions are renewed before they expire so you can keep taking your medications.

Remember, communication is key. Always ask your questions and express your concerns. Your pharmacist is here to help you navigate through the world of pharmacy and healthcare, so feel free to reach out and ask for advice or clarification. Here's to making your pharmacy experience as seamless and positive as possible!

18.3: Practical Problem-Solving Tips

Dealing with pharmacy issues can be stressful and confusing, but don't worry! I'm here to share some practical solutions for those times when things don't go quite as planned. Here are some solutions to common issues that come up at the pharmacy:

"My medication is not in stock."
If the medication you need isn't currently available at the pharmacy, they can always order it for arrival the next business day. If you need it immediately, don't worry about making multiple calls yourself. The pharmacy will handle locating it for you. Most chains can search stock for pharmacies within a certain radius of their location, typically 20 miles. If they are able to locate it, they can arrange for the prescription to be transferred to the location that has it in stock, given you are open to pick it up at another location. This ensures you get your medication without unnecessary delays or added stress. (See Chapter 1.7 for more details)

"My medication is on a backorder."
Discovering that your medication is on backorder can be stressful, but don't worry; your pharmacy team is equipped to handle this for you. They'll start by searching nearby locations within their pharmacy chain to see if another location has your medication in stock. If they do, they'll work with the other location to transfer your prescription over, provided you agree to pick up the medication at the alternative location.

If this search for stock doesn't find another location, your pharmacy team can contact your doctor to inform them of the backorder status. If you are open to it, your pharmacy team can also ask your doctor if they would like to consider providing you with an alternative medication and provide suggestions for alternative medications.

Suppose you or your doctor do not want to consider alternative medications. In that case, your pharmacy team can place your medication on perpetual ordering, which means keeping it on order until the medication is available. This will put you at the front of the line, and your prescription will be automatically filled once the medication is available and shipped to the store for dispensing.

It's important to understand that a pharmacy's ability to check stock at other pharmacies is limited within the same chain. If you are considering trying a different pharmacy chain due to availability issues, you would have to make those calls yourself, as the pharmacy cannot search the stock of other chains. However, your active participation in the process, such as following up with your doctor, not only speeds up the process but also serves as an additional reminder to your doctor's office. Remember, collaboration between you, your pharmacist, and your healthcare provider is key to effectively dealing with backorders. (See Chapter 1.8 for more details)

"My controlled medication is out of stock, and I need it."
The management of controlled or narcotic medications comes with additional regulations, especially when stock issues arise. It's important to know that, as a patient, you cannot directly call pharmacies to check stock levels for these types of medications. There are strict regulations about these medications, and pharmacies have to follow policies surrounding safety and security. Instead, the pharmacy that has your medication should be able to help you. First, they can search for the stock of your medication within their pharmacy chain. If located, due to the controlled nature of these drugs, a new prescription needs to be issued by your doctor's office to the location that has your medication, and they must also cancel the current prescription. Your pharmacy can either inform your doctor's office directly of the new pharmacy location where they can send your new prescription, or you can share that information with your doctor's office after your pharmacy has informed you. This process ensures that the handling of controlled substances is done safely and in accordance with legal requirements while also helping to maintain your treatment continuity without unnecessary delays. (See Chapter 1.7 for more details)

"My medication frequency changed, and now it's too early to fill, according to my insurance."
If you have run out of your medication due to changes in how often and how much you are taking it, contact your pharmacy. They can work with

your insurance company to get a change in therapy override, allowing you to fill your medication sooner based on the new directions you are taking. This typically involves getting a new prescription from your doctor reflecting the new directions.

"I can't find my medication."

If your medication has gone missing, whether misplaced, lost, or stolen, don't worry; your pharmacy team has a solution. Reach out to your pharmacist, and they'll help you figure out what to do next. If you have remaining refills, your insurance might allow for a lost or stolen medication override. If not, you always have the option to pay out-of-pocket and still receive your medication. In this case, ask your pharmacy team if they have a discount program that can help you with cost. If you no longer have refills, your pharmacy team can reach out and ask for a renewal, but you might have to reach out directly to your doctor to provide details as to why you need another renewal. For controlled substances, a police report might be needed.

"I need an extra supply of my medication because I am traveling out of the country for an extended period."

Many insurance plans allow for a vacation override, which allows you to get an extra refill of your medications for long trips. Let your insurance company and pharmacy know ahead of time about your trip. With enough notice, your pharmacy team can secure a vacation override. Depending on your insurance, you might have to provide your travel itinerary. If your insurance doesn't offer this, ask your pharmacist about other options, such as paying out of pocket for the additional supply.

"My prescription isn't ready when I go to pick it up."

Always check the status of your medications before heading over to the pharmacy for pick-up. You can do this by checking your app or simply calling the pharmacy to confirm your medications are ready. If you arrive and your medications aren't ready yet, ask if you can wait while they work on it. Your pharmacy team can often expedite a prescription to the front of the line if you ask to wait for it, getting the medication ready for pick-up in 15 minutes or less. Depending on the current staff, you may have to get back in line and wait your turn to ring out once your medication is ready.

If delays happen often, ask about the best times to submit and pick up prescriptions to avoid the rush.

"I was charged the wrong amount for my medication."
If you believe there's been an error in the amount you were charged for your medication, call or visit your pharmacy and bring your receipt. Let the Pharmacist know what doesn't add up, and they'll work to troubleshoot it with you. Be prepared to provide insurance cards, coupons, and discounts that should have been applied. Corrections to the price can usually be made directly at the pharmacy if they're within the insurance billing period, which is typically 14 days or less from when the medication was filled. Should more time have passed, reaching out to your insurance company directly might still get you a refund. (See Chapter 4.7 for more information)

"My insurance refuses to cover my prescription."
Insurance issues are common but fixable. Talk to your pharmacist; they can check if the problem is a prior authorization requirement, a formulary change, or simply an administrative error. They can explain why your medication isn't covered and review potential solutions with you. (See Chapter 4 for more information).

"I forgot to refill my prescription, and now I'm out of medication."
If you're out of refills, a quick call or visit to your pharmacy can usually get you a new refill as quickly as 15 minutes or less if you decide to wait in the pharmacy. Suppose you don't have any refills and need your medication immediately; ask your pharmacist about a hold-over supply. This is usually a three-day emergency supply, only available for essential medications while the pharmacy waits for a new prescription from your doctor's office. (See Chapter 15.4 for more details)

"I received the wrong medication."
Your safety is of utmost importance. If you think there's been a mix-up, bring the medication back to your pharmacy without taking any doses. If you're not able to do so, you can also call and ask for the pharmacist. They can check your prescription and verify the medication. There's a

chance that the manufacturer may have been different, and you, indeed, still have the correct medication on hand. If any errors were indeed made, your pharmacist will correct any errors found immediately and inform you of the next steps.

"I'm not sure how to properly use my new medication."
Whether it's an inhaler, insulin injections, or a new topical cream, your pharmacist is available to counsel you, as well as provide hands-on demonstrations and clear instructions. Don't hesitate to ask. (See Chapter 3.1 for more information on medication administration)

"My child refuses to take their medication due to the taste."
Many liquid medications offer flavoring options. Certain tablets can be crushed, while some capsules can be opened and sprinkled on apple sauce. Talk to your pharmacist about these concerns, and they can provide tips on making medication time less stressful for both you and your child. (See Chapter 10.3 for more details)

"My prescription requires special handling or storage, and I'm not sure how to manage it."
Medications like biologics or certain eye drops may need refrigeration or special care. A good rule of thumb is to store the medication the same way you received it from the pharmacy. Storage requirements are also often printed on the medication package itself. If you're not sure and need additional guidance, call or visit your pharmacy, and they can provide detailed instructions on how to store, handle, and administer the medication. Don't hesitate to ask for a demonstration or clarification.

"I'm worried about interactions between my prescription medications and over-the-counter (OTC) products."
If you are taking medications, always inform your pharmacist about any OTC products, supplements, or herbal remedies you plan to take prior to starting them. Your pharmacist can review your entire medication list to identify potential interactions and offer safe alternatives if needed.

"I accidentally dropped my medication down the sink/toilet."
Accidents happen, but it's important to handle them safely. If you lose medication in a way that it cannot be recovered or used, contact your pharmacy. Depending on the medication, they can help you get an emergency refill. For controlled substances, you'll likely need to report the incident to your doctor for further guidance. (See Chapter 1.4 for more information)

Pharmacy problems can be frustrating, but they often have straightforward solutions. Your pharmacy team is here to support you and ensure you get the medications you need with as little hassle as possible. No matter how big or small your questions or concerns are, don't be afraid to ask for help.

FURTHER READING FOR CHAPTER 18:
PHARMACY FAQS AND TROUBLESHOOTING

American Pharmacists Association (APhA)
For a detailed understanding of pharmacy policies and procedures, and to access a wide range of frequently asked questions answered by pharmacy professionals, visit the American Pharmacists Association.
Available at: www.pharmacist.com.

Pharmacy Times
Explore articles and resources that provide answers to common pharmacy questions and offer practical tips for problem-solving in the pharmacy setting at Pharmacy Times.
Available at: www.pharmacytimes.com.

National Association of Boards of Pharmacy (NABP)
Gain insight into pharmacy policies and learn about the regulatory guidelines that shape these practices by visiting the National Association of Boards of Pharmacy.
Available at: www.nabp.pharmacy.

CONCLUSION

If you're here at the end of this book, I just want to say thank you. You've made space to learn, to care, and to figure things out—even when it's not always easy.

This book wasn't about perfect routines or quick fixes. It was built to offer steady support for the real-life moments that show up: a fever in the middle of the night, a stomach that won't settle, a lingering headache that needs something simple and safe.

You now have something to come back to. Not just for the remedies—but for the reassurance that you're not alone in this.

Here's what you've got in your hands:

- Practical guidance on how medications work—and how to use them with confidence
- Herbal and natural support options that are actually grounded in research
- At-home care ideas that don't need fancy tools or special training
- Gentle reminders for how to take care of your people and yourself
- Tips for navigating the bigger stuff—insurance, side effects, medication safety, and more

No one expects you to have all the answers. This book is here for those "What now?" moments—the ones that happen when someone's not feeling well and you're trying to figure out the next right step.

Use what's helpful. Come back when you need to. And if something doesn't feel right, know it's always okay to reach out for more support.

You're doing the best you can with what you've got. And that's enough.

Thanks for letting me be part of it.

ACKNOWLEDGMENTS

Before we close this chapter, I just want to say thank you. This book didn't come together on its own, and so many people helped make it happen.

To the moms, patients, and caregivers who've shared your stories and questions with me over the years—you're the reason this book exists. Your honesty, your strength, and the way you keep showing up inspired every single page.

To my family and friends—especially my husband and daughters—you are everything. Thank you for cheering me on, keeping me grounded, and giving me the space to write. I couldn't have done this without you.

And finally—to you. Thank you for letting me walk beside you. Writing this felt like chatting with a friend, and I hope it brought you a little more confidence, a little more calm, and maybe even a few smiles when you needed them most.

Here's to the love you give, the strength you show, and the quiet, powerful ways you keep supporting yourself and your loved ones.

ABOUT THE AUTHOR

Hi—I'm Rhowela Albana Friel. I'm a pharmacist, a mom of two girls, a wife, and someone who's spent years helping families make sense of healthcare.

Pharmacy has always been part of my story. My mom was a pharmacist, my dad a family doctor, and I grew up in the Philippines watching them care for people through our little family-owned pharmacy. Some of my earliest memories are of sitting behind the counter, watching people come in with questions and leave with real help. That's what healthcare has always meant to me: showing up when it matters most.

After moving to the U.S. at 13, I kept following that path. I started working at CVS after high school, became a pharmacist, and grew into roles that let me support both patients and pharmacy teams—as a Pharmacy Manager, a Supervisor, and later a District Manager for specialty pharmacies serving underserved communities. These days, I'm a Clinical Pharmacist working with state programs to improve access to essential medications.

But nothing has shaped me more than becoming a mom. My girls have taught me more than any textbook ever could. They're the reason I started writing—because I know how hard it can be to figure things out while still being the one everyone counts on.

This book came from that place. From wanting to offer something real and helpful. From knowing what it's like to be tired, unsure, and still trying your best.

I don't have all the answers—but I'll keep show-ing up with what I do know, and what I've learned through both my career and this messy, beautiful, everyday life.

There's more ahead—more books, more support, and more real talk for real life. I'm so glad you're here.

ADDITIONAL RESOURCES

Thank you again for picking up this book. I hope it brought you a little more clarity, a little less stress, and maybe even a few deep breaths when you needed them most.

If you're wondering what comes next—I've got you.

You can find me at rhowelaafriel.com, where I've gathered everything I've created (and am still creat-ing) to help you feel steady, supported, and pre-pared—without the overwhelm.

Here's what you'll find there:

- Books – A look at what I've already writ-ten and what's coming next. Each one is built to walk alongside you.

- The Blog – Stories, tips, and encourage-ment—some personal, some practical—all written like we're chatting over coffee.

- Recommended Products – A no-stress roundup of the things I actually use and love, all in one place.

- The Shop – Simple tools like checklists, guides, and downloads to make the every-day feel a little easier.

- Contact – Have a question or just want to connect? I'd love to hear from you.

The site's easy to explore—so stop by anytime. I'll be there, building more resources to help you take care of yourself and the people you love.

www.ingramcontent.com/pod-product-compliance
Lightning Source LLC
Chambersburg PA
CBHW050050230526
45470CB00004B/1473